Oncology
for the
House Officer

Oncology
for the
House Officer

Joseph F. O'Donnell, M.D.
Associate Professor of Clinical Medicine
Associate Dean for Student Affairs
Dartmouth Medical School
Hanover, New Hampshire
Chief, Medical Oncology
VA Hospital
White River Junction, Vermont

Christopher T. Coughlin, M.D.
Professor of Clinical Medicine (Radiation Therapy)
Dartmouth Medical School
Hanover, New Hampshire

Paul J. LeMarbre, M.D.
Clinical Associate Professor of Medicine
Medical College of Wisconsin
Milwaukee, Wisconsin

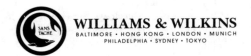

WILLIAMS & WILKINS
BALTIMORE · HONG KONG · LONDON · MUNICH
PHILADELPHIA · SYDNEY · TOKYO

Editor: Michael G. Fisher
Managing Editor: Carol Eckhart
Designer: Dan Pfisferer
Illustration Planner: Ray Lowman
Production Coordinator: Adèle Boyd-Lanham

Copyright © 1992
Williams & Wilkins
428 East Preston Street
Baltimore, MD 21202 USA

Accurate indications, adverse reactions, and dosage schedules for drugs are provided in this book, but it is possible that they may change. The reader is urged to review the package information data of the manufacturers of the medications mentioned.

Printed in the United States of America

Library of Congress Cataloging-in-Publication Data

Oncology for the house officer / Joseph F. O'Donnell, Christopher T. Coughlin, Paul J. LeMarbre.
    p.   cm.
    Includes index.
    ISBN 0-683-06626-9
    1. Cancer. 2. Oncology. I. O'Donnell, Joseph F. II. Coughlin, Christopher T. III. LeMarbre, Paul J.
    RC261.0475 1991
    616.99′4—dc20

    91-14095
    CIP

91 92 93 94
1 2 3 4 5 6 7 8 9 10

It is widely felt that there is no more trying period in the development of the physician than the housestaff training period. One of the most complicated and often most emotionally draining aspects can be the care of patients with cancer. They can be so sick from both their disease and the toxic therapies, as well as have surrounding them all the terrible images and myths that our society has associated with cancer.

This book is meant to be an introduction—a "survival manual" containing some pertinent facts and explaining some key concepts about cancer. There are many excellent, detailed texts available which can supply the background to fill in where this book is necessarily superficial. But even these texts are having difficulty keeping pace with the rapid developments in the field of cancer medicine. Our last chapter on ways to access new data through the use of the computer, the library and the continuously updated data bases suggests the ways we feel are best to keep current in the field.

Until the AIDS epidemic, there was no disease more feared by the U.S. public than cancer. Yet tremendous gains in the understanding and treatment of cancer have already taken place. The current progress in molecular genetics, cell biology and immunology have put us closer to the center of understanding the puzzle of cancer than ever before. We still have a long way to go, but we stand at the dawn of an era of diagnosis, treatment and most of all, prevention, that we never even dreamed about twenty years ago.

We hope that this book will give you, the future health providers of our population, an accurate and hopeful overview of the "cancer problem."

Joseph F. O'Donnell, M.D.

About the Book

This text is a multi-authored collection from the oncology faculty of Dartmouth Medical School and the Norris Cotton Cancer Center. The concepts in the book and the sequence in which they appear come from a course in the pathobiology of cancer that we give to our medical students at Dartmouth.

The book is divided into specific chapters dealing with aspects of cancer medicine and aimed to give a general overview of each to the busy house officer. As such, though, if one wishes to quickly look up information about a specific cancer or a specific situation, the organization of the book may make this more difficult. For example, if one wished to find information about breast cancer, statistics would be given in Chapter 1, epidemiology in Chapter 2, prevention and screening in Chapters 4 and 5, diagnostic principles in Chapter 6, some "pearls" about the disease in Chapter 19, and finally, the way to find the "latest" information literally updated monthly, in Chapter 20.

A very useful companion book in the series currently in production is *Case Studies in Oncology* by Dr. Maurie Markman, Vice Chairman, Department of Medicine, Memorial Sloan-Kettering Cancer Center. This book will "fill out" and complement our book by giving specific case examples with documentation of the management strategies through appropriate literature references.

We hope you find this book useful and helpful and would appreciate any constructive feedback.

Contributors

Susan M. Bauer Boyarsky, R.N., M.S., O.C.N.
Instructor in Clinical Medicine, Dartmouth Medical School, Hanover, New Hampshire

Thomas A. Colacchio, M.D.
Associate Professor of Surgery, Dartmouth Medical School, Hanover, New Hampshire

Christopher T. Coughlin, M.D.
Professor of Clinical Medicine (Radiation Therapy), Dartmouth Medical School, Hanover, New Hampshire

Gerald Gehr, M.D.
Chief of Medical Service, VA Hospital
Adjunct Assistant Professor of Medicine, Dartmouth Medical School, Hanover, New Hampshire

Michael P. Grace, M.D.
Assistant Professor of Clinical Medicine, Dartmouth Medical School, Hanover, New Hampshire

Paul J. LeMarbre, M.D.
Clinical Associate Professor of Medicine, Medical College of Wisconsin, Milwaukee, Wisconsin

L. Herbert Maurer, M.D.
Professor of Medicine, Dartmouth Medical School, Hanover, New Hampshire

Kenneth R. Meehan, M.D.
Instructor in Clinical Medicine, Dartmouth Medical School, Hanover, New Hampshire

Letha E. Mills, M.D.
Associate Professor of Clinical Medicine, Dartmouth Medical School, Hanover, New Hampshire

William A. Nelson, Ph.D.
Associate Professor of Clinical Psychiatry
Director, Section of Medical Humanities, Dartmouth Medical School,
Hanover, New Hampshire

Joseph F. O'Donnell, M.D.
Associate Professor of Clinical Medicine and
Associate Dean for Student Affairs, Dartmouth Medical School, Hanover,
New Hampshire
Chief, Medical Oncology, VA Hospital, White River Junction, Vermont

Susan J. Scown
Editor, Norris Cotton Cancer Center, Dartmouth-Hitchcock Medical
Center, Hanover, New Hampshire

Christopher W. Seidler, M.D.
Instructor in Clinical Medicine, Dartmouth Medical School, Hanover,
New Hampshire

Contents

Chapter 1

Introduction to Cancer Medicine

In the minds of many people, the diagnosis of cancer is often equated with interminable suffering and death, yet today almost 50% of cancer patients are surviving five years and the majority of them are "cured" by current approaches. Many more patients have significant extensions of their useful lives or improvements of the quality of their remaining lives. The future prospects from the better understanding of the basic sciences of cancer biology have never been more hopeful.

At the bicentennial of Harvard Medical School, Dr. Daniel Federman stated:

"We stand at the dawn of an era of prevention, of diagnosis and of treatment that our forebears never even imagined."

The field of cancer medicine is undergoing an exciting and explosive growth. You as house officers will see and experience some advances we never could even imagine.

DEFINITION

Cancer is difficult to define, but the authors like the following definition, compiled from various sources, best:

"Cancer is a popular generic term for malignant neoplasms (new growths or tumors), a great group of diseases of unknown and probably multiple causes, occurring in all human and animal populations and arising in all tissues composed of potentially dividing cells. The basic characteristic of cancer is the transmissible abnormality of cells

that is manifested by reduced control over growth and function leading to serious adverse effects on the host through invasive growth and metastases."

Cancer is derived from the Greek word "karkinos," meaning crab. It was felt that the large veins surrounding breast masses looked like the claws of a crab.

Some call cancer a "disease of civilization," but actually it dates back more than one million years. Traces of bone cancer have been seen in an anthropoid skeleton in Java that is over one million years old. Also, there are references in early Hindu and Egyptian writings, and mummies from 2500 BC have also shown evidence of bone cancer.

KEY FACTS ABOUT CANCER

Every year the American Cancer Society publishes a full set of data. House officers either should receive in their mail (for free) the yearly update published in the January-February issue of *CA—A Journal for Physicians* or may call their local ACS office to receive a copy of this or the yearly updated *Cancer Facts and Figures*. These sources detail such information as trends, survival rates, new cases, and deaths, both for the nation as a whole and by state.

Here are some "facts" that the authors feel should be readily available to housestaff:

1. **Cancer is the second leading cause of death in the U.S.** There were 1,040,000 new cases and 510,000 deaths in 1990. Heart disease ranks first, causing 38% of the deaths in the U.S., while cancer causes about 20%. (In perspective, though, about as many people die of sudden cardiac death as die from cancer.)

2. **Cancer is the second leading cause of death in children,** causing about 5% of deaths while accidents cause about 20% of deaths. Cancer kills more children than any other disease, though.

3. **Americans have about a one in four chance of developing cancer and a one in six chance of dying from it**. Cancer directly affects three out of four families.

4. **Overall, the five year survival rate for a person with cancer has climbed from one in five in the 1930's to one in three in the 1960's.** Forty-nine percent of those diagnosed in 1989 with cancer will, in fact, be alive five years later. There are over five million people alive today with a diagnosis of cancer, and over three million of them have survived for five years or more.

5. In 1988, the National Cancer Institute published the 36-year trends in cancer mortality (1950–85) (Journal of the National Cancer Institute 80(1):8, 1988). Table 1.1A lists the percentage changes by age group.

All ages had decreased death rates from cancer except those over 55. When lung cancer is excluded, only the 85 + age group has an increase, and that by only 0.1% as seen in Table 1.1B.

These advances occurred despite a 37% overall increased cancer incidence for whites (23% if lung cancer is excluded). Data for blacks are not available for the whole period from 1950–85, but *recent data show that cancer rates have been increasing even more rapidly in blacks.*

For the first time in recent years, lung cancer incidence rates decreased in men last year, but unfortunately, lung cancer incidence rates in women are the fastest rising of all cancer incidence rates in the U.S.

Table 1.1A
36-Year Trends in Cancer Mortality (1950–85) (Rates/100,000 Persons)

Age	Percent Change (All Cases)
0–4	− 67.3
5–14	− 47.0
15–24	− 37.6
25–34	− 34.7
35–44	− 24.6
45–54	− 3.1
55–64	12.6
65–74	22.0
75–84	12.4
85 +	10.5
All ages	9.1

Table 1.1B
36-Year Trends in Cancer Mortality (1950–85)

Age	Percent Change (All Sites Excluding Lung)
0–4	−67.0
5–14	−46.2
15–24	−36.1
25–34	−35.4
35–44	−32.9
45–54	−23.0
55–64	−14.8
65–74	−7.9
75–84	−8.1
85+	0.1
All ages	−13.3

Table 1.2
Incidence of Cancer in U.S. Population (for 1989)

Community Population	Cancer Cases Under Care	New Cases	Will Develop Cancer	Will Die of Cancer
1,000	5	3	280	180
10,000	52	33	2,800	1,800
100,000	525	333	28,000	18,000

6. Even though these figures depict cancer as a common disease, **in a given individual at a given age, cancer is an uncommon finding.** This is illustrated in Table 1.2 (adapted from *ACS Facts & Figures*, 1989, p. 15.).

In general, primary care physicians rarely diagnose a "new" patient with cancer. Physicians with a practice of 1,000 patients would see only three new cases per year. Many patients, however, come to see their physicians because they are afraid that their symptoms may represent cancer.

7. Just as in the practice of medicine, **the practice of oncology has dramatically shifted toward emphasis on care provided in ambulatory**

care situations. If a house officer only cares for inpatients with cancer, he or she will see a disproportionately high number of patients either very sick from the cancer or the therapies or in the process of dying. Today, most chemotherapy and virtually all radiation therapy is done on an out-patient basis. House officers should elect an outpatient experience in oncology, if available, for a good overview of what an oncologist really does.

8. **Cancer accounts for more than 2 million hospitalizations annually in the U.S.** (about 5.5% of all hospitalizations). Cancer ranks third behind pregnancy/delivery and heart disease as a cause of hospitalization, but in terms of bed-days in hospital, it is second only to heart disease.

The most common cancers causing death in the U.S. by age group are listed in Tables 1.3 and 1.4.

9. **By the year 2000, cancer will rank second as a cause of death worldwide.** The current incidence and death rates for the 10 most common cancers in the less industrialized countries of the world are listed in Table 1.5.

Table 1.3
Mortality for the Five Leading Cancer Sites for Males by Age Group

All Ages	Under 15	15–34
Lung	Leukemia	Leukemia
Colon & rectum	Brain & CNS	Skin
Prostate	Non-Hodgkin's lymphomas	Brain & CNS
Pancreas	Connective tissue	Non-Hodgkin's lymphomas
Leukemia	Bone disease	Hodgkin's

35–54	55–74	75 +
Lung	Lung	Lung
Colon & rectum	Colon & rectum	Prostate
Brain & CNS	Prostate	Colon & rectum
Non-Hodgkin's lymphomas	Pancreas	Pancreas
Skin	Stomach	Bladder

Table 1.4
Mortality for the Five Leading Cancer Sites for Females
by Age Group

All Ages	Under 15	15–34	35–54
Breast	Leukemia	Breast	Breast
Lung	Brain & CNS	Leukemia	Lung
Colon & rectum	Bone	Uterus	Colon & rectum
Pancreas	Bladder	Brain & CNS	Uterus
Ovary	Non-Hodgkin's lymphomas	Non-Hodgkin's lymphomas	Ovary

55–74	75 +
Lung	Colon & rectum
Breast	Breast
Colon & rectum	Lung
Ovary	Pancreas
Pancreas	Ovary

Table 1.5
Deaths and New Cases of the Most Frequent Cancers in the
"Third" World (New Cases and Deaths Are Listed per 100,000
Population.)

Site	New Cases	Deaths
Stomach	336	280
Esophagus	254	231
Lung	206	187
Liver	192	174
Cervix	370	154
Colon & rectum	183	108
Mouth & pharynx	272	101
Breast	224	97
Lymphoma	122	81
Leukemia	106	81

Because of the heavy smoking habits now occurring in these countries, lung cancer will soon be the leading cause of cancer death just as it is in the developed countries of the world.

10. Trends in five-year survivals are presented in Table 1.6 (adapted from *ACS Facts & Figures*, 1989, p. 17.).

Table 1.6
5-Year Survival Percentages by Cancer Site

	Whites		*Blacks*	
	1960–63	*1979–84*	*1960–63*	*1979–84*
All Sites	39%	50%	27%	37%
Oral cavity & pharynx	45	54	*	31
Esophagus	4	7	1	5
Stomach	11	16	8	17
Colon	43	54	34	49
Rectum	38	52	27	34
Liver	2	3	*	5
Pancreas	1	3	1	5
Larynx	53	66	*	55
Lung & bronchus	8	13	5	11
Melanoma	60	80	*	61
Breast (females)	63	75	46	62
Cervix uteri	58	67	47	59
Corpus uteri	73	83	31	42
Ovary	32	37	32	36
Prostate	50	73	35	60
Testis	63	91	*	82
Urinary bladder	53	77	24	57
Kidney & renal pelvis	37	51	38	53
Brain & nervous system	18	23	19	31
Thyroid gland	83	93	*	95
Hodgkin's disease	40	74	*	69
Non-Hodgkin's lymphoma	31	49	*	49
Multiple myeloma	12	24	*	29
Leukemia	14	32	*	27

*Data not available.

IS THERE A CANCER EPIDEMIC?

The answer is no. Because of the aging of the population, the cancer rate per 100,000 people is only slightly higher than in the past. Death rates are rising more dramatically in non-white populations, though. Even so, if smoking-related cancers are separated out, the rates are actually *lower* now than in the past.

Dramatic gains have been made in younger people. Figure 1.1 shows that most of the death rates per 100,000 people have remained constant, but steadily decreasing rates have been seen since 1966 in those under 45.

As can be seen in Table 1.7, many of the other causes of death have declined dramatically. Thus, cancer appears to cause more deaths.

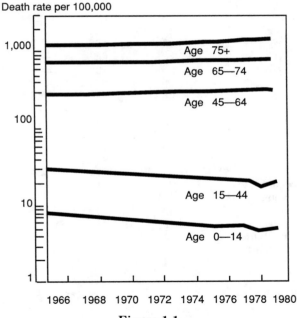

Figure 1.1

Table 1.7
Changes in Age-adjusted Mortality Rates (Per 100,000 People) Between 1960 and 1985, U.S., All Races

Cause	Sex	1960	1985	% Change
Cancer	M	143	164	+ 15
	F	111	111	0
Heart disease	M	376	248	− 34
	F	206	127	− 38
Stroke	M	85	35	− 59
	F	75	30	− 60
Pneumonia/flu	M	35	18	− 49
	F	22	10	− 55
Accidents	M	74	52	− 30
	F	27	19	− 30
All non-cancer causes	M	806	552	− 32
	F	479	298	− 38

CANCER CONTROL OBJECTIVES FOR THE YEAR 2000

The National Cancer Institute has published a set of objectives with the goal of reducing the cancer mortality rate by 50% in the year 2000.

The goals are presented in Table 1.8. The major categories are primary and secondary prevention (screening), discussed in Chapters 4 and 5, and application of the latest "state-of-the-art" treatments, discussed in Chapter 20. Treatment for cancer continues to evolve. The developments in cancer medicine are coming at a rapid pace, and the literature is voluminous. One of the best ways to stay current with the "best" treatment options for your patients is to consult the data base "PDQ," which is updated monthly. Alternatively, the house officer can call 1-800-4-CANCER and receive up-to-date, annotated searches of the cancer literature or call ONCOLINE (a free service of Roche Laboratories) at 1-800-443-6673; Virginia residents call collect 703-391-7829.

Table 1.9 details the relative contributions of each prevention goal to the overall estimate of reduction in the mortality rates.

These goals are achievable, but to reach them will require the coordinated efforts of physicians, nurses, cancer educators, and organizations

Table 1.8
Cancer Control Objectives

Action	Target	Year 2000 Objectives
Prevention	Smoking	Reduce the percentage of adults who smoke from 34% to 15% or less. Reduce the percentage of youths who smoke by age 20 from 36% to 15% or less.
	Diet	Reduce average consumption of fat from 37–38% to 30% or less of total calories. Increase average consumption of fiber from 8–12 to 20–30 g/day.
Screening	Breast	Increase the percentage of women ages 50–70 who have an annual physical breast examination coupled with mammography to 80% from 45% for physical examination alone and 15% for mammography.
	Cervix	Increase the percentage of women who have a Pap smear every 3 years to 90% from 79% (ages 20–39) and to 80% from 57% (ages 40–70).
Treatment	Transfer of research results to practice	Increase adoption of state-of-the-art treatment.

like the American Cancer Society, the insurance industry, and the government.

ORGANIZATION OF CANCER CARE IN THE UNITED STATES

The central organization for the care of the cancer patient in the United States is the National Cancer Institute (NCI). The NCI is one of seventeen divisions of the National Institutes of Health (NIH). The NCI sets goals, policies, and priorities for the nation's fight against cancer. It is divided into five major subdivisions: the divisions of cancer etiology, cancer biology and diagnosis, cancer treatment, cancer prevention and control, and the extramural program, which oversees the work done away

Table 1.9

Estimated Reduction in Cancer Mortality Rate by Year 2000 by Prevention, Screening, and Treatment

Objective	Method	Estimated Reduction in Mortality Rate
Prevention	Smoking	
	Reduction in adult smoking prevalence to 16%	
	a) if achieved in year 2000	8%
	b) if achieved in year 1990	15%
	Diet	8%
	Fat reduction to 25% of total calories	
	Fiber increase to 20–30 g/day	
Screening	Achievement of objectives in Table 1.8	3%
Treatment	Application of current state-of-the-art treatment for specific cancer sites	
	a) with no future changes in state-of-the-art therapy	10%
	b) with current trend in state-of-the-art survival (0.5% per year, all sites) maintained	14%
	c) with accelerated gains in state-of-the-art treatment (1.5% per year, all sites)	26%
Total range of mortality reduction in percent		25–50%

from the primary locations in Bethesda and Frederick, Maryland. The leaders of the Cancer Institute are advised by the National Cancer Advisory Board consisting of eleven nonvoting, *ex-officio* members (the heads of major governmental agencies dealing with health) and eighteen members appointed by the President. Twelve of the eighteen are scientific leaders and the remaining six come from the public and include leaders in health policy, law, economics, and management.

The NCI has established regional "cancer centers" all over the country. The mission of these cancer centers is: 1) to provide the most up-to-date, state-of-the-art treatment for the patient with cancer utilizing all the modalities that are proven to be effective; 2) to educate both the public and the professional communities about the developments in cancer ranging from prevention and early detection to the latest advances in treatment and rehabilitation; and 3) to continue to expand the knowledge base and understanding by doing both basic science and clinical research.

Many types of medical professionals work together to care for the patient with cancer. Physicians who deal primarily with cancer are called oncologists, which is derived from the Greek word "onkos," meaning tumor. There are three major types of oncologists.

Surgeons were actually the first oncologists. Surgery is still the most effective therapy against cancer, and virtually every subdiscipline of surgery involves care of cancer patients. Cancer can be a substantial part of the practice of the general surgeons. Today, multiple post-residency training programs focus on oncology, give special training in understanding the natural history of cancer, and teach the principles and use of effective therapies against it. Currently, there is not a board certification in the subspecialty of surgical oncology, but at some point there may be. In addition to the general surgeon, much of the work of some surgical subspecialists involves oncology. In urology, otolaryngology, neurosurgery, plastic surgery, and orthopedics, there are clinical practitioners who focus their practice and research predominantly on cancer. Another surgical subspecialty that devotes a great deal of attention to oncology is gynecology, and specialists in gynecologic oncology are trained in the special techniques needed to manage ovarian, uterine, and cervical cancer. Gynecologic oncologists are also trained in the principles of chemotherapy, and they often administer these agents to their patients. In addition, in anesthesia a great many physicians are now involved in the field of chronic pain control and they deal with many cancer patients.

Radiation oncology is another discipline involved with the care of the cancer patient, using radiation as the prime modality of therapy. As with the other types of oncologists, in order to give effective "total care" to the patient, radiation oncologists must know a great deal about the biology and natural history of cancer as well as other modalities used for treatment. Radiation oncology is often underemphasized in the medical school curriculum. House officers may not get a view of this specialty. Next to surgery, radiation is the most effective curative modality for cancer and it is also extremely effective in palliation of symptoms. Radiation oncologists are able to get a great deal of satisfaction because of the effectiveness of their therapy for their patients with cancer. There is a three-year training program after an internship which may be in surgery, medicine, or transitional. Radiation oncology is currently an undersubscribed profession, and there are many new developments in radiation biology, including the use of radiation combined with other therapies. These are very exciting for the future effectiveness of this field.

Medical oncology is one of the newest of the medical subspecialties. It deals primarily with the use of chemotherapeutic agents in the management of cancer, but the medical oncologist must also have a sound knowledge base in the other disciplines involved with cancer therapy. Medical oncologists are now also beginning to utilize the new and exciting biological response modifier therapies. Trainees enter medical oncology after three years of medicine. There is a two-year fellowship period. Currently, one may take boards for certification in both hematology and oncology (which are often combined) by spending three years in training (18 months of these three years must be involved in direct patient care). This will soon change to a required four years. There are projected to be about 4,900 board-certified medical oncologists in the United States in the year 1990. There are currently 159 programs listed in the AMA's 1988–89 *Directory of Graduate Medical Education Programs.*

Many other health professionals are involved with the field of oncology. Others include nurses, epidemiologists, "basic" scientists, social workers, chaplains, primary care physicians, health educators, radiation physicists, radiation therapists, radiation biologists, and psychiatrists. In Chapter 17 some specific suggestions for the house officer to maximize the "care" of his or her patient with cancer by interactions with these professionals are discussed.

Cancer touches every medical specialty. It is such a common diagnosis that encounters with patients will occur frequently in just about any medical practice. There are several points that a house officer should remember.

1. Though there is much still be to done, there is very much that can be done now to help the cancer patient conquer sometimes and cope always with the disease.

2. The effort against cancer is a team effort. Hopefully, at your institution there will be team meetings involving all of the professionals who see the cancer patient. If formal team meetings about the cancer patient do occur, take an active part. Ask questions of all the professionals involved.

3. One type of meeting that often occurs in a medical center is called a Tumor Board. In this meeting, experts representing various disciplines gather to discuss the management of a specific patient. The house officers should use this as a tremendous opportunity to learn from this collection of combined wisdom and, during such a conference when a patient is presented, should be asking himself or herself, "What would I do now?" and how does it agree or disagree with what the experts say. Be active in these conferences.

4. Finally, cancer is a community, and even more, a family disease. Cancer affects all members of the family. It has a great impact on the community, from the work place, to the church, to the schools and other social organizations.

Housestaff should be aware of the volunteer organizations. These are discussed in Chapter 17.

CANCER PROTOCOLS

The optimal treatments for many types of cancer and for cancers of different stages are still being defined. Part of the process of trying to advance the progress against cancer is through the use of treatment protocols. House officers often find these cumbersome. Decisions seem to be taken away by a rigid, already defined treatment system that, at times, seems "cookbook."

One can learn a great deal from protocols, though. Here are some of the author's suggestions. Protocols usually have the following sections:

1. Introduction and scientific background
2. Objectives
3. Selection of patients (eligibility)
4. Study design
5. Treatment programs
6. Procedures in the event of toxicity
7. Required clinical and laboratory data
8. Criteria for evaluating the effect of treatment
9. Statistical considerations
10. Specifics on therapy
11. Informed consent

12. Data forms
13. References

These may be in a different order, or have different headings, but usually a protocol contains these elements. The introduction (and reference section) usually contains a capsule summary of the "state-of-the-art" of a particular therapy against a particular tumor, and gives the rationale for the protocol. The "objectives" section discusses what the protocol is trying to prove. The sections on design and statistics offer useful reviews of quantitative methods for clinical research. The therapy sections and specifics of therapy cover the drugs used, their pharmacology and toxicities (and how to avoid the latter). The house officer should review in his or her own mind the elements of informed consent—what to tell the patient about the risks and benefits of the program and the alternatives.

One of the most crucial elements of a protocol is the way results are evaluated. The house officer should carefully measure and record lesion size and results of appropriate laboratory tests. Is the therapy working? How do I know or can I tell? By actively thinking about the protocol, one can learn much about the disease, and protocols can be good learning tools instead of just "cookbooks."

SOME TERMINOLOGY

Protocols are divided into three major types:

Phase I studies evaluate toxicity and dose-schedule. They are usually done in patients who have "failed" other therapies. Any response of the tumor is an added bonus.

Phase II studies evaluate a specific dose or schedule against a specific tumor.

Phase III studies compare the current "best" therapy against the experimental treatment. For some tumors, there is no "best" treatment and the effects are measured against appropriate controls. Phase III studies may also identify equally effective regimens that may have less toxicity.

The optimal evaluation of a treatment would be against a tumor one can measure and see if it responds by shrinking in size. It is not always possible to find measurable tumors. When a tumor is measurable, there are several types of responses defined as follows:

Complete response = complete disappearance of all evidence of the tumor.

Partial response = decrease by 50% in the volume of tumor.

No response = no change, or a shrinkage of less than 50%.

Progression = growth of the tumor (or appearance of new lesions) in spite of therapy.

EVALUATING A REPORT ON CANCER THERAPY

There are literally thousands of articles written each year about various treatments for various cancers. Chapter 20 discusses how to access these. How do you know if what you read is applicable to your patient? The author's suggestions are as follows: You must read the title and abstract carefully, but do not base judgments on whether to use the therapy on these alone. Always carefully review the methods of patient selection, exclusion, staging, evaluation of response, and toxicity.

Important questions to ask include:

1. What kinds of patients were selected for the trial? How do they compare to the patient I'm considering giving this therapy? (Parameters to consider include stage of disease, performance status, prior therapy, and co-morbid illnesses.)

2. How "much" therapy did the patients in the trial get? What are dosing levels and time intervals? How was dose modified for toxicity and what type of toxicity was seen? Could this degree of toxicity be tolerated in my patient?

3. What were the criteria for response? It is best to use the objective criteria defined above for measurable lesions (i.e., complete response, partial response, etc.). Were subjective criteria used? If so, did the tumor really get smaller and/or did the patient live longer and better?

4. How did the authors report the trial? What was the denominator for response reporting? Was it entered patients, evaluable patients, adequately treated patients? How did they define the latter? How did they handle their patients who were lost to follow-up? Are they presenting too "rosy" a picture by excluding all but their "best" patients from the analysis?

5. What did they compare their therapy against? Historical controls (which are always a hazard) or were there appropriately matched controls?

The house officer should review reports of cancer therapy trials with seasoned staff oncologists. What seems "too good to be true" often is. A dramatic illustration of reporting the same data and getting two different interpretations is given in an article by Baar and Tannock, in *Journal of Clinical Oncology* (7:969–78, 1989). They give two presentations of the *same* fictitious data on combination chemotherapy for "metastatic cancer of the great toe." One illustration (by the "esteemed" authors "Apples and Oranges") shows the "CABOOM" regimen to be very effective, while the same data (this time by the equally "esteemed" "Prose and Conns") shows "CABOOM" to be ineffective. These tongue-in-cheek articles make unforgettable points about the cancer literature and are worth review.

Chapter 2

Cancer Epidemiology

Epidemiology is the study of the distribution of disease in populations, and the factors that determine the distribution. By its nature, epidemiology cannot prove causation; it can only provide clues. These clues may be important to discern etiology, to identify high risk groups, and to apply appropriate preventive measures.

This chapter will list the types of cancer alphabetically, give some descriptive statistics about them, and identify various risk factors. By necessity, this list will not be all-inclusive, and it will only identify the most common cancers to which the house officer should be exposed and their most important risk factors.

The concept of "risk" needs some comment. There is a great deal of confusion about "risk," and in general, people find it difficult to put risk into perspective. There are many reasons for this, including the emotional overlay the "risk" of cancer has, the legal and political ramifications of risk and how the media often portrays risk with a certain sensationalism. Furthermore, most people cannot even fathom the concepts of small levels of risk. Does being in that building with asbestos insulation mean I'll get cancer? What happens if I eat that apple that might have alar on it?

Although some risks haven't been quantified yet, and some not even fathomed, we do have good ideas about some "risks." They can range from the 100% incidence of cancer in those who have the gene for familial polyposis coli to the small increase in incidence for those who live in granite houses and who are exposed to low level radiation. There are risks we can and should do something about. These will be discussed in Chapter 4.

In taking and recording the medical history, the house officer should list the risks. He or she should work with the patients and their families to change what is changeable in regard to risk. This should be an integral part of the plan that is developed to care for the patient.

Biliary Tract Cancer (includes cancer of gallbladder and biliary ducts)

1. Accounts for less than 1% of cancer in the United States, but 5% in Latin America and Israel. In the U.S., these cancers are seen more frequently in Native Americans and Hispanics.

2. In the U.S. there are:
   1.0 cases/100,000 in white men
   1.8 cases/100,000 in white women

The highest incidence is in New Mexico, where there are:

   2.5 cases/100,000 in Hispanic men
   9.2 cases/100,000 in Hispanic women
   22.3 cases/100,000 in Native American women
   5.9 cases/100,000 in Native American men

3. The incidence increases with age. These cancers are seen more commonly in women.

4. Most people who get these cancers have gallstones, but the converse (i.e. most people with stones get cancer) is not true.

5. In Asia, biliary cancer is associated with infestation by the liver fluke, *Clonorchis*. Biliary cancer is also seen in increased incidence in typhoid carriers and in workers in the rubber industry.

Bladder Cancer

1. Common in northeastern United States. Very common in Egypt— related to schistosomiasis there.

2. In the U.S., the incidence is:
   17.8/100,000 in white males
   4.7/100,000 in white females
   9.4/100,000 in black males
   3.2/100,000 in black females

3. There were 50,200 cases and 9,500 deaths in 1991.

Risks:

1. Smoking increases risk by two times compared to the general population.

2. Possibly saccharin and coffee.

3. Working in rubber, leather, or dye industry, and asphalt, coal tar, and pitch workers. There are increased risks in painters, truck drivers, auto mechanics, drill press operators, blacksmiths, hairdressers, and petroleum processors.

4. Associated with use of Cytoxan (cyclophosphamide).

5. Renal pelvis cancer associated with renal papillary necrosis, stones, and analgesic abuse.

6. Associated with *Schistosomiasis haematobium* where that is prevalent (produces squamous cell carcinoma).

Breast Cancer

1. The most common cancer in women. 175,000 cases and 44,800 deaths in the U.S. in 1991.

2. There is a small increase in incidence.

3. The disease is seen more frequently in North America and Northern Europe and less frequently in Asia. Breast cancer is more often seen in urban locations and in women of higher socioeconomic status.

4. In U.S., the incidence in white women is 64.6/100,000 and 50.4/100,000 in black women. A woman born in the U.S. has a 12% risk of developing breast cancer in her lifetime.

Risk factors include:

1. Female sex—breast cancer does occur rarely in males, though.

2. Age.

3. Prior breast cancer in the opposite breast.

4. Family history—all women who have breast cancer in their family, especially the first degree relatives of breast cancer patients, are at increased risk. Those in whom the breast cancer in relatives occurred

before menopause are at greater risk. The greatest risk occurs in women whose first degree relatives had bilateral breast cancer. This is illustrated by the following table:

Family History

First Degree Relative Developed Cancer	Patient's Risk	Estimated Lifetime Risk for Patient
Premenopausally	3.1 ×*	28%
Postmenopausally	1.5 ×*	14%
Bilateral breast cancer	5.4 ×*	49%
Premenopausally	8.8 ×*	79%
Postmenopausally	4.0 ×*	36%

*General population.

Factors 2, 3, and 4 are considered the major risk factors putting women at high risk. Other factors include:

5. "Fibrocystic disease." 50% of women have this. Are they all then at increased risk? It turns out that 70% of these women have pure cysts filled with fluid and do not seem to be at increased risk, while 30% of women with this condition have hyperplastic (hypercellular) changes. This 30% is made up of 26% with typical benign appearing hyperplasia, and 4% with what is called atypical hyperplasia. This latter type of fibrocystic disease is associated with subsequent development of cancer and should be considered a MAJOR RISK FACTOR. The trouble is that one can only tell that atypical hyperplasia exists by doing a biopsy. Physical exam and mammography don't tell the types of fibrocystic disease apart.

If in your breast physical exam, you are unsure about nodularity you feel, you should refer the woman to a physician experienced in breast diagnosis for a careful exam and possible aspiration for cytology. You should also strongly consider a mammogram, especially in women over 35 years of age. If a prior biopsy has come back with the diagnosis "atypical hyperplasia," that woman should be considered at high risk.

The "so called" minor risk factors include:

6. History of radiation exposure to the breast (e.g. through mammography).

7. Early onset of menarche and late menopause.

8. Age at first child's birth. The earlier in life a pregnancy and birth occurs, the lower the risk for that mother. Breast cancer rates are also increased for those women who have their first child when they are over thirty.

9. Obesity. Some try to link breast cancer to fat in the diet but this relationship is not clear. In addition to increased risk in general, cancers in obese women may be being detected at later stages because of difficulty with examination.

10. Alcohol use seems to increase risk.

11. Diethylstibestrol use during pregnancy, which was popular to prevent "morning sickness," may increase risk of breast cancer in the mother and does increase the incidence of clear cell adenocarcinoma of the vagina in the daughters.

    The use of estrogens at menopause probably increases risk slightly. The risk is greatest for unopposed estrogens and some compounds are more strongly associated than others. A recent cohort study from Sweden (*N Engl J Med*: 321:293–297, 1989) showed a slight increase in risk, especially when estradiol was used. In this study in contrast to other studies, the addition of progestins did not seem to lessen the risk. There are many studies about this subject, and the definitive answer has not yet been obtained. On the contrary, the benefits of postmenopausal estrogen replacement are well known. Much work still needs to be done to define the safest doses and type of hormone replacement.

12. Breast cancer is seen more frequently in women with ovarian cancer, endometrial cancer, and colon cancer.

13. Breast cancer is seen more frequently in men with Klinefelter's syndrome.

    Despite this long list of risk factors, many women (estimated 75%) seem to have only female sex and age as their personal "risks." This behooves us to try to offer tests for early diagnosis (e.g. mammography) to *all* our women patients in the appropriate age groups.

Central Nervous System Tumors

1. Increased incidence seen in Israel, Northern Europe, and especially Switzerland. Decreased in Asia and Eastern Europe.

2. In the U.S.
   6.3 cases/100,000 in white men
   4.1 cases/100,000 in white women
   3.7 cases/100,000 in black men
   3.3 cases/100,000 in black women

3. Seen more frequently in people of higher socioeconomic status.

4. There is an increased incidence of gliomas and acoustic neuromas in neurofibromatosis.

5. Incidence is increased in rubber workers.

Cervical Cancer

1. Highest rates in Appalachia in U.S., Colombia, and Brazil; low in Israel and U.S. whites.

2. In the U.S., the rates are:
   13.8/100,000 in white females
   30.4/100,000 in black females

3. Invasive cancer is decreasing by 2%/year but *in situ* cancer is rising.

4. There were 13,000 cases and 4,500 deaths in 1991.

Risks:

1. Frequent sexual contact with multiple partners ("a disease of prostitutes").

2. Poor hygiene.

3. Smoking (moderate increase).

4. Human papilloma virus (HPV, especially types 16 and 18), and herpes simplex virus II seem related to cervical cancer. Exactly how is not clear. Laboratory studies have strongly implicated HPV as an etiologic agent, but epidemiologic studies are inconsistent.

5. More cervical cancer is seen among women who use oral contraceptives and less among those who use barrier methods.

6. Foods high in vitamin A *may* protect. Vitamin C and folate *may* also protect.

7. Clear cell adenocarcinoma is seen in daughters of women who used DES in pregnancy.

Colorectal Cancer

1. Increased in U.S. (especially the northeast), Canada, and Scotland. Decreased in central Europe, Japan, and Africa.

2. Directly proportional to socioeconomic status (but weak association). Also, more commonly seen in urban areas, but rural clusters are seen (e.g. the southeast corner of Nebraska where the high incidence seems related to genetic factors).

3. In the U.S. the incidence is:

25 cases/100,000 (colon) 13.6 cases/100,000 (rectum)	For white males
22.2 cases/100,000 (colon) 8.3 cases/100,000 (rectum)	For white females
21.4 cases/100,000 (colon) 11.6 cases/100,000 (rectum)	For black males
22.0 cases/100,000 (colon) 6.8 cases/100,000 (rectum)	For black females

   There were 157,000 cases and 60,500 deaths in the U.S. in 1991.

4. There is a rapid change in migrants from one culture to another.

Risk Factors:

1. Age—93% occur after 50.

2. Family history increases risk by 3–4 times over the general population, but there are rare familial syndromes that greatly increase risk:

   Familial polyposis coli—100% incidence in affected members (autosomal dominant).
   Gardner's syndrome—there is an increased risk of colon cancer in this syndrome of epidermal cysts, subcutaneous fibromas, osteomas, and adenomas of the G. I. tract.
   Peutz-Jeghers syndrome—there is a slight increase of cancer in this syndrome which is characterized by intestinal polyps and oral mucosal pigmentation.

3. Colon polyps. There are 3 types of polyps—villous, adenomatous, and hyperplastic. The first two types increase the risk of colon cancer and removal of the polyps decreases risk. 10% of people older than 50 have polyps. There have been attempts to find clues to identify these "polyp

formers." Some suggest that people with skin tags in the axilla and neck to be at increased risk, but this is controversial.

4. There is ever stronger data accumulating on the role of dietary fat. At the present time, this dietary constituent seems more important than fiber and the intake of certain vitamins like A, C, and E. Calcium in the diet may also play a role in protection from cancer, but this is by no means clear. Beer consumption may be associated with rectal cancer.

5. Acquired diseases like ulcerative colitis and Crohn's disease increase risk. For ulcerative colitis, risk is associated with the degree of bowel involvement, the disease activity, and the length of time of the disease. A person with active and extensive ulcerative colitis for 10 years has a $10\times$ greater risk of developing colon cancer.

6. Colon cancer is also increased in people with acromegaly, Barrett's esophagus, and breast, endometrial, and ovarian cancer.

7. Colon cancer is increased in asbestos workers, shoe workers, and machinists.

8. Patients who have had ureterosigmoidostomies are at increased risk.

Endometrial Cancer (Corpus Uteri)

1. More common in U.S. whites, Canada, and northern Europe ($10\times$). Decreased in Japan, Israel, and Singapore. In the U.S. more common in the midwest.

2. Weakly associated with socioeconomic status.

3. In the U.S. there are:
   17.9 cases/100,000 white females
   10.0 cases/100,000 black females

4. There were 33,000 cases and 5,500 deaths in 1991.

Risks:

1. Inversely related to parity.

2. Directly related to age of menopause.

3. Obesity.

4. Diabetes.

5. High blood pressure.

These five risks have something to do with the hormonal state that leads to low parity and late menopause, and which occurs in overweight women prone to diabetes and hypertension.

6. Increased five times in family members of patients.

7. Increased in women with breast and/or ovarian and/or colon cancer.

8. Use of estrogens at menopause—6–7× increased risk. This is proportional to duration and dose of estrogens and decreased with use of combination estrogen/progestin replacement.

Esophageal Cancer

1. There were 10,900 cases and 9,800 deaths in the U.S. in 1991.

2. There is a very high incidence in Iran, China, and the Kazakhastan region of the USSR east of the Caspian Sea. There are also very high rates in Britain, France, and the coastal regions of South Carolina in the U.S.—all of which seem related to alcohol preparation and consumption.

3. The incidence in the U.S. is:
   3.6 cases/100,000 in white males
   1.1 cases/100,000 in white females
   13.9 cases/100,000 in black males
   3.3 cases/100,000 in black females

4. The 5 year survival is only 3%.

5. It is seen in men of lower socioeconomic status and in more commonly in urban environments.

Risks:

1. Directly related to alcohol and tobacco use. Each alone is a risk, but in combination, they are synergistic.

2. The incidence is increased in patients with achalasia and a history of lye strictures. It is felt that the stricture prevents food from passing quickly into the stomach and allows carcinogens in the diet to contact the surface epithelium.

3. Carcinoma of the cervical esophagus is seen as increased incidence in patients with severe iron deficiency producing an esophageal web (Plummer Vinson syndrome).

4. People with poor dentition have increased incidence.

5. Diets low in vitamins A, C, and possibly riboflavin have been incriminated, but this link is by no means clear.

6. In Japan, the habit of men consuming the hot food and sake has been suggested as a possible link. Women may only eat after the men have finished.

7. There is a rare inherited disease called tylosis which is associated with hyperkeratosis of the palms and soles and an association with esophageal cancer.

8. Barrett's esophagus increases the risk of adenocarcinoma of the gastroesophageal junction.

Gastric

1. Worldwide this is the most common cancer.

2. In the U.S. the incidence has been decreasing dramatically since the turn of the century. The reasons are not clear, but some suggest that the greatest achievement in cancer was the invention of the refrigerator replacing smoking, pickling, and other modes of preserving food. The U.S. rates have dropped 60% since the 1930's and now are among the lowest in the world.

3. Rates in Japan, Chile, Colombia, Singapore, Costa Rica, and Iceland remain very high.

4. There were 23,800 cases and 13,400 deaths in 1991 in the U.S.

5. It is associated with low socioeconomic status.

Risks:

1. Pernicious anemia increases risk $5 \times$.

2. Atrophic gastritis increases risk $3 \times$.

3. Smoking is associated with cancer in the cardia region.

4. Seen after radiation (e.g. Hiroshima, Nagasaki).

5. 2–3× increase in relatives

6. Seen more frequently in farmers, fishermen, coal miners, and asbestos workers.

7. The role of diet is unclear, but nitrosamines seem important. The most widely accepted theory is that certain diets predispose to nitrosation of amines in foods providing endogenous nitrosamines and other carcinogens (some formed by the process of cooking, others by food preservation techniques). This latter situation was especially true in the past when "pickling" and "smoking" were important ways to preserve food. This process of nitrosation may be inhibited by vitamins C or E or other antioxidants.

8. There are some reports of increase in incidence after partial gastrectomies. This is controversial and not clearly established.

Head and Neck Cancer

1. Seen most commonly in urban areas in the U.S., Brazil, India, and Spain. Low incidence in Norway, Iceland, and Japan.

2. Incidence increasing in women.

3. Reverse correlation with socioeconomic status.

4. Seen in women in factories in Southeastern U.S. (believed due to chewing tobacco), and in people who chew betel nut or quid in India. Nasopharyngeal cancer seen in furniture makers in North Carolina (due to the glues?), and in Cantonese Chinese exposed to E.B. virus.

5. In the U.S. for laryngeal cancer, the incidence is:
8.3/100,000 for white males
1.3/100,000 for white females
12.1/100,000 for black males
1.9/100,000 for black females

For cancer of the mouth and throat, the incidence is:

16.8/100,000 for white males
6.0/100,000 for white females

19.3/100,000 for black males
7.0/100,000 for black females

Risks:

1. Smoking (10× above nonsmokers).

2. Alcohol (3× above baseline—note, the combination of smoking and alcohol synergistic).

3. Chewing tobacco.

4. Workers with asbestos exposure, nickel, petroleum, and metal workers are also at slightly increased risk. Nasopharyngeal cancer (see above) also seen in increased incidence in pottery, linoleum makers, battery makers, and wood, leather, and shoe workers.

5. There is a small increased incidence of tongue cancer in those patients with syphilis who have had a chancre on their tongue. Also, there is a risk of pharyngeal cancer in patients with severe prolonged iron deficiency, especially if a web developed.

6. Squamous cell cancer of the mouth is being seen in patients with AIDS, leading to more speculation for a possible viral etiology in these immunocompromised patients.

7. Pipe smokers are prone to lip cancer. This is also seen in those with heavy sun exposure (e.g. farmers, sailors, and other outdoors oriented people).

Leukemia

1. There were 11,600 cases and 7,600 deaths of granulocytic leukemia and 11,700 cases and 5,200 deaths of lymphocytic leukemia in 1991 (this includes acute and chronic types).

2. Accounts for 5% of cancer in the U.S., but 45% of cancer in children. Increases with age, but there is an early peak of acute lymphocytic leukemia.

3. A.L.L. is the "usual" type of leukemia in childhood, but all types occur. In Ankara, Turkey, AMML (acute myelomonocytic leukemia) accounts for 40% of cases in young children.

4. Chronic lymphocytic leukemia (CLL) is rare in Japan. Men have $2\times$ greater risk of CLL than women.

5. Directly proportional to socioeconomic status.

Risks:

1. Exposure to benzene, chemotherapeutic (alkylating) agents, and chloramphenicol.

2. Related directly to radiation exposure (except CLL).

3. Increased in Down's syndrome, Bloom's syndrome, and Fanconi's syndrome.

4. The only *definite* human virus causing cancer is HTLV-1, which causes T-cell leukemia/lymphoma. Other viruses are suspected.

5. There are "clusters" reported frequently, but the relationship of leukemia to such things as chemical dumps is not clear (e.g. the Love Canal in Buffalo).

6. Leukemia occurs in patients who have the hematologic diseases called myelodysplastic syndromes. There are 5 subcategories of these.

7. CLL is the one type most likely to be seen in families.

8. There may be a slight increase of leukemia in smokers.

Liver Cancer (Hepatoma)

1. Worldwide a very important tumor. Highest incidence seen in the Orient, Central Europe, and Africa. In the U.S., it is not common and accounts for only 0.6% of cancers.

2. In the U.S., the incidence rates are:
   2.3/100,000 for white males
   1.1/100,000 for white females
   4.6/100,000 for black males
   1.2/100,000 for black females

Risks:

1. Aflatoxin exposure. Aflatoxin B is a substance produced by certain strains of *Aspergillus flavus*. It has been shown to be one of the most

potent hepatotoxins known. It has been found to contaminate many food products (especially peanuts and grain) and probably acts as an initiating agent.

2. Hepatitis B. This may act more as a promoter— causing initiated cells (e.g. cells damaged by exposure to aflatoxin) to divide and progress to a cancer. The hepatitis B vaccine may have a profound effect in decreasing the incidence of this disease. Hepatitis B virus infection seems to increase the rates of liver cancer most in regions with the highest aflatoxin levels.

3. It is seen in people with cirrhotic livers, especially cirrhosis due to hemachromatosis.

4. Increased incidence is seen in those exposed to anabolic steroids, arsenic, and vinyl chloride (tanners, smelters, vintners, and plastic workers).

5. Thoratrast, which was used as an angiographic agent, may be associated with angiosarcomas of the liver.

6. There are several cases of liver tumors seen after use of methotrexate.

Lung Cancer

1. Will soon become the most common cancer worldwide. Smoking is increasingly being taken up by people in the less developed countries, and soon, they will join the industrialized countries with lung cancer as the leading cause of cancer death.

2. There were 161,000 cases and 143,000 deaths in 1991 (about 15 deaths/ hour) in the U.S.

3. In the U.S., it is the leading cause of cancer death in males and has just surpassed breast cancer as leading cause of cancer death in females. Incidence has tripled in both males and females in last 25 years, but incidence in males is beginning to drop.

4. Age peak 65 for male; 75 for female (rare <40).

5. Economic loss >$3 billion/year.

6. 7-fold difference in worldwide incidence in males from highest to lowest country.

7. In U.S., incidence is increased in urban areas, lower socioeconomic groups, areas with greater percentages of non-white residents, and areas with transportation, paper, chemical, and petroleum industries. Incidence is increasing more rapidly in non-white population.

8. In U.S. the incidence is:
   57.0/100,000 for white males
   12.1/100,000 for white females
   74.5/100,000 for black males
   12.2/100,000 for black females

Risks:

1. Smoking is clearly implicated, by both retrospective and prospective studies.

   a. Risk is proportional to number of cigarettes smoked, depth of inhalation, and age at which smoking began. Cigar and pipe smoking are less dangerous for lung cancer than cigarette smoking.

   b. Despite clear knowledge that smoking is dangerous, too many American continue to smoke. The percentage of male smokers has dropped, however, from 52% of the population in 1964 to 31% in 1987, and in females from 34% in 1964 to 27% in 1987. However, with elimination of smoking, lung cancer would be virtually eliminated. (Counting other diseases, 450,000 deaths/year are now attributed to cigarettes.)

   c. Cigarette smoke is a mixture of over 2,000 chemicals. It has been called the "perfect carcinogen." It even contains radiation! The exact chemical(s) responsible for lung cancer is/are unknown.

   d. Safer cigarettes are being developed, but at the present time, it can be said that *no* cigarette is truly safe. Filter cigarettes are better, and low tar may be better, but people seem to smoke more when smoking low tar/low nicotine, and may in fact be exposed to *more* dangerous substances.

   e. Heavy smokers are addicted to nicotine. Much of smoking behavior and reputed beneficial effects can be attributed to prevention of withdrawal symptoms.

   f. Smoking is clearly related to development of squamous cell, small cell, and large cell carcinoma. Also, there is increased risk of adenocarcinoma in smokers, although this subtype is the one *least* associated with smoking.

2. Air pollution, especially "reducing" type, i.e., London type, pollution— incidence *may* be *slightly* increased. One chemical measured is 3, 4-benzpyrene, and exposure to atmosphere with 10 ng/m^3 benzpyrene is equivalent to smoking one cigarette a day.

3. Asbestos exposure: With heavy exposure, if you also smoke, there is a 92 times increased risk of dying of lung cancer (8 times increased risk if workers do not smoke).

4. Radon. See Chapter 4.

5. Rarer causes (occupational exposures): Nickel refining (ore and use), radiation exposures, especially uranium mining, chromates (ore miners, glass workers), bis(chloromethyl) ether, mustard gas, arsenic, and iron oxide (factory workers, metal grinders). Occupations: miners, chemical workers, vintners, asbestos users, textile users, insulation workers, tanners, smelters, glass and pottery workers, coal tar and pitch workers, iron foundry workers, electrolysis workers, radiologists, newspaper workers (black ink).

6. Host factors:

   a. In general, lung cancer incidence is increased 2-4 times in families of patients. In the future, we may be better able to predict who is genetically susceptible to certain carcinogens.

   b. "Scars" in the lungs secondary to other diseases, e.g., TB, sarcoid, pulmonary fibrosis, etc., may be the site of the development of a carcinoma.

7. Role of vitamin A: There is some evidence that vitamin A may protect against lung cancer. This is under active study.

Lymphomas (Hodgkin's Disease)

1. Hodgkin's disease makes up about 25% of the cases in the U.S. of malignant lymphoma (7,400 cases in the U.S. in 1991).

2. The incidence is:
3.5/100,000 in white males

2.4/100,000 in white females
3.0/100,000 in black males
1.2/100,000 in black females

3. The incidence is highest in the U.S. white population (also northern Europeans) and lower in the Orient and Hawaii.

4. It is one of the most common cancers of young adults, but rare in children under 5. There are 2 age peaks—one in the early 20's and another higher peak in the late 70's. In Japan, only the second peak is seen. Some suggest because of these peaks that there may be more than one disease process responsible.

5. There have been several clusters reported, but the speculation of an infectious etiology has not yet been proved.

6. The risk is proportional to educational level.

7. The risk is greater in smaller families and in people with prior tonsillectomies.

8. Siblings of patients have a seven times increased risk.

9. Hodgkin's disease is seen now in patients with AIDS and other immunodeficiency states (e.g. ataxia telangiectasia).

Lymphomas (Non-Hodgkin's)

1. Makes up 75% of lymphomas in the U.S. (37,200 cases in the U.S. in 1991).

2. The incidence is:
10.7/100,000 in white males
8.2/100,000 in white females
7.2/100,000 in black males
4.7/100,000 in black females

3. It is found to be increased in patients with both congenital and acquired immunodeficiency diseases. It is also seen as a second malignancy after successful treatment for Hodgkin's disease.

4. Non-Hodgkin's lymphomas may run in families.

5. One subtype—Burkitt's lymphomas, found in Africa—is strongly associated with Epstein-Barr virus, but whether this is causal or a paraphenomenon is not clear.

6. The first human retrovirus proved to cause a malignancy is HTLV-I. This causes a T-cell malignancy that is found in the Caribbean, Southern Japan, Africa, and recently in the United States.

7. Rarely, patients treated with diphenylhydantoin may develop a "pseudolymphoma" and even more rarely, a frank malignant lymphoma.

8. Chemists have a higher risk of lymphoma, but the specific chemicals implicated are not known.

Melanoma

1. Next to lung cancer in women, this is the fastest rising cancer in the U.S. This rise is believed due to lifestyle changes, with increased outdoors leisure time in the sun, and clothing changes allowing more exposure.

2. Seen in white people of higher socioeconomic status. Incidence increases in U.S. as latitude decreases (proportional to sun exposure).

3. There were 32,000 cases and 8,500 deaths in 1991.

4. High incidence also seen in Australia—felt to be due to the English, Scottish, Irish migrants with fair skin.

Risks:

1. Sun exposure.

2. History of blistering sunburns especially in childhood.

3. Fair complexion (blue eyes, red or blond hair).

4. There is a relatively newly recognized syndrome called the "dysplastic nevus syndrome" in which affected people have unusual moles (usually many large ones). These may and often do progress to melanoma. There is an outstanding atlas of these dysplastic nevi which all house officers should review and keep (*N Engl J Med* 312:91, 1985).

5. Those with congenital giant hairy nevi are at increased risk.

6. It is suggested that pigmented lesions in area of possible trauma (e.g. soles of the feet or belt buckle area) may be at risk.

7. Tanning salons (see Chapter 4).

Multiple Myeloma

1. This is the 13th most common type of cancer in the U.S. in blacks, and the 19th in whites.

2. In the U.S., the incidence rates are:
   4.3/100,000 in white males
   3.0/100,000 in white females
   9.6/100,000 in black males
   6.7/100,000 in black females

3. There were 12,300 cases and 9,100 deaths in 1991.

4. Rates rising—not known why.

Risks:

1. Radiation exposure (e.g. almost 40 years after Hiroshima and Nagasaki increased myeloma seen).

2. Work with lead vapors, plastics industry, farming, wood, leather and petrochemical workers.

3. Siblings of patients have a slightly increased risk.

4. Myeloma has been seen after long courses of lupus, rheumatoid arthritis, and scleroderma.

Ovarian Cancer

1. Higher incidence in northern Europe, Canada, U.S. whites. Decreased in Japan, Spain, and Cuba.

2. In the U.S., the incidence is:
   12.3/100,000 in white females
   9.2/100,000 in black females

3. There were 20,700 cases, and 12,500 deaths in 1991.

4. The incidence appears to be decreasing somewhat in younger women, while increasing in older women.

5. Moderately associated with socioeconomic status.

Risks:

1. Nulliparous women are twice as likely to develop ovarian cancer.

2. Radiation exposure (Hiroshima and Nagasaki) produced a two times increase in risk, but diagnostic and therapeutic radiation have not been shown to increase risk.

3. Asbestos exposure; also possibly talc use.

4. Women with breast and/or endometrial cancer have an increased risk.

5. Women with Peutz-Jeghers syndrome (intestinal polyposis and oral mucosal pigmentation) are reported to have a 5–14% chance of ovarian cancer.

6. Use of birth control pills *may* protect women from ovarian cancer.

Pancreatic Cancer

1. Has risen greater than 30% between 1951 and 1978 in the U.S.

2. Seen more frequently in Hawaiians, Native Americans, and people of Jewish ancestry. It is 10 × more common in Switzerland. The incidence is decreased in Seventh Day Adventists and Mormons.

3. Inversely related to socioeconomic status.

4. In the U.S., the incidence is:
9.3/100,000 in white males
5.5/100,000 in white females
13.2/100,000 in black males
7.5/100,000 in black females

5. There were 28,200 cases and 25,200 deaths in 1991.

Risks:

1. Smoking (2 × general population).

2. Alcohol—possible.

3. Diabetes gives slightly increased risk.

4. Seen more frequently in chemists, pharmacists, and coke and gas plant workers.

5. There is a great deal of speculation on the linkage to diet, but the exact mechanism and/or dietary culprit is unknown. One frequently cited contributor is dietary fat, and animal models corroborate this—most likely unsaturated fat. Coffee has been suspected, but the data on this is very controversial, and most experts currently do not believe this is a risk.

6. Islet cell tumors may be inherited as part of the MEN I (Wermer's) syndrome.

Prostate Cancer

1. Prostate cancer is said to be the cancer men die "with" rather than "of." The following table displays the percentage of men at various ages discovered to have foci of prostate cancer at autopsy.

Age	Foci of Cancer Found at Autopsy
<50	0%
50–59	29.2%
60–69	30.2%
70–79	40.1%
80–89	70.6%

Still, far too many men die of prostate cancer, and the course of the disease can be very painful.

2. There were 122,000 cases and 32,000 deaths in 1991.

3. In the U.S., the incidence is:
39.7/100,000 in white males
67.4/100,000 in black males

4. The incidence in the U.S. is rising, especially in the north central states. There is a low incidence in Japan.

5. It is inversely proportional to socioeconomic status.

Risks:

1. Family history (3×).

2. Rubber industry, and possibly working with lead.

3. Some speculation about fat in the diet, but very controversial.

Renal Cancer (Hypernephroma)

1. High in Scandinavia, Canada, and the U.S.; low in Asia and Africa.

2. There were 25,300 cases and 10,600 deaths in the U.S. in 1991.

3. In the U.S., the incidence is:
7.1/100,000 in white males
3.4/100,000 in white females
6.4/100,000 in black males
3.2/100,000 in black females

Risks:

1. Cigarette smoking (slight).

2. Asbestos exposure and possibly petroleum workers.

3. Possibly associated with obesity in women.

4. There are some families with renal cancer. These have been associated with chromosomal abnormalities (3–11, 3–8 translocations).

Testicular Cancer

1. Most common type of solid tumor in 20–34 year old males. Second most common cancer in U.S. in 35–39 age group; third in 15–19 year olds.

2. Low rate in blacks. In the U.S., incidence is:
3.6/100,000 in whites
0.8/100,000 in blacks

3. 6,100 cases, but only 375 deaths. A real treatment "success" story.

Risks:

1. Cryptorchidism (undescended testes). There is a 10–40 times increased risk. Seminomas are most frequently associated. If the testes is in the

inguinal canal, there is a less than 1% chance, but if intraabdominal, the risk approaches 5%. The cancer occurs in the contralateral testis (i.e. not the undescended one) in 20–25% of cases.

2. Possibly linked to DES use by the mother during pregnancy (but most experts feel this is not likely).

Thyroid Cancer

1. In the U.S. the incidence rates are:
   2.0/100,000 for white males
   5.0/100,000 for white females
   1.0/100,000 for black males
   3.0/100,000 for black females

2. There were 12,400 cases and 1,000 deaths in 1991.

3. Seen in people of higher socioeconomic status.

Risks:

1. Radiation to the neck—often for benign conditions like acne, tinea capitis, or blocked eustachian tubes.

2. Medullary carcinoma has both a sporadic and an inherited form. The latter is inherited in an autosomal dominant fashion, and may be either alone or part of the MEN-II syndrome (Sipple's syndrome).

Chapter 3

Brief Review of Tumor Biology

The present is a very exciting time in the history of cancer medicine. The discoveries—especially in the fields of molecular genetics, cell biology, and immunology—have brought scientists closer to understanding the basic mechanisms of cancer than ever before. Yet, each new insight poses multiple new questions to be asked and technologies to be developed to try to answer them. We are still very far from understanding many of the mysteries of cancer, but these new discoveries are coming at a very rapid pace.

It is very difficult for anyone, even experts in specialized areas of tumor biology, to stay abreast of all the new developments. Important articles on understanding cancer appear in almost each new issue of journals like *Nature* and *Science.* Many of these discoveries do not have immediate effects on the care of our patients, but without doubt, they will change how oncology is practiced in the future.

The house officer needs to be aware of this excitement and of the potential for significant new changes in diagnosis, therapy, and especially in the basic understanding of cancer. The information in textbooks, medical school lecture notes, and even journal articles may be rapidly superseded by new discoveries. The authors feel that the electronic data bases discussed in Chapter 20 hold the potential for doctors to stay abreast of the most recent developments. These are updated monthly and are the most up-to-date source for new developments.

Each year, the American Society of Hematology (ASH) and the American Society of Clinical Oncology (ASCO) have education sessions and publish education booklets on new developments. House officers should ask their attendings in hematology and oncology to share this information. Also, each year, *JAMA* publishes a brief description of some of the important new developments in the various fields of medicine.

There are many detailed texts that deal with the aspects of cancer biology that follow in this chapter. The authors will try to make brief points about the topics that may be of interest in the present management of patients, or of possible significant future potential.

CARCINOGENESIS

The following diagram summarizes the carcinogenic process.

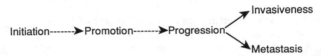

It is clear that carcinogenesis is a multistep process, and that often the steps represent alterations in the genome or the expression of genes. For simplicity, the process can be divided into two steps: *Initiation* and *Promotion*.

Initiation involves irreversible alteration of the genome by substances known as initiators. Initiators are mutagens and as such are detected by the Ames test, which tests chemicals for their ability to mutate bacteria. Initiators are likely present all around us and may act in single exposures. There is no apparent threshold dose and the effects of multiple exposures are additive.

Promoters act after initiators to "promote" the development of a cancer from the growth of the "initiated" cells. Promoters by themselves are not carcinogenic (initiators are). Chronic exposure is required and since they are not mutagens, tests like the Ames assay fail to detect them.

The classic sequence is as follows:

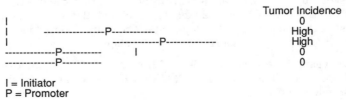

Promotion may involve things like:

a. Continuing to smoke (cigarette smoke is called the "perfect" carcinogen because it contains both initiators and promoters)

b. Diet (high fat diets are suspected)

c. Infections (like hepatitis B, which causes growth of hepatocytes and clonal expansion of initiated cells)

d. Medications (estrogens for example in liver cell adenomas, some of which may progress to carcinomas)

Promotion is likely to involve a multistep process, and it is likely that some of the steps are reversible. Much work is being done to try to develop "anti-promoters" to inhibit the progression of initiated cells to frank cancer, and many of the "chemoprevention" trials may be thought of in this way:

Does a low fat diet decrease chances of developing breast cancer?

Does the use of vitamin A supplements prevent skin or lung cancer?

Do calcium, vitamin A, C, or E supplements inhibit the development of colon polyps and subsequent colon cancer?

Will hepatitis vaccine prevent liver cancer?

The important messages for the house officer are:

1. Initiators are all around us. Some are being identified and our exposures limited by the government testing agencies.

2. Promoters may be much more manageable. Many promoters may be things we do to ourselves that stimulate cell turnover (e.g. diet, smoking, infections, medications).

3. Anti-promoters are being developed and are very promising.

4. Before irreversible changes occur, compounds may be developed that induce differentiation back to the "normal" state, e.g. cis-retinoic acid has been given in some cases of acute promyelocytic leukemia with some evidence of differentiation of the blasts. Cis-retinoic acid has also been shown to make oral and cervical preneoplastic lesions regress.

ONCOGENES AND ANTIONCOGENES

One of the most exciting areas of cancer research is that of oncogenes. The field of retroviral oncogenesis and chemical carcinogenesis have come together and a new understanding of the basic mechanisms underlying cancer is developing. The following definitions come from the lectures of George Sorenson, M.D., Professor of Pathology at Dartmouth Medical School.

Some definitions:

Viral oncogene (V-onc)—A gene found in some retroviruses (RNA tumor viruses) that can cause neoplastic transformation in target cells.

Proto-oncogene (or cellular oncogene or C-onc)—A type of gene probably found in all of our genomes. It can be picked up by a virus to form a viral oncogene, or altered by many factors to become a transforming gene which can cause a cell to become malignant. The proto-oncogene likely has functions that deal with growth and differentiation of normal cells, but when changed, it can cause a normal cell to become malignant.

Anti-oncogene—A newly described type of gene whose product inhibits growth. Loss of such a gene may allow for abnormal, uncontrolled growth. These genes are recessively inherited.

More than 60 oncogenes have been identified to date and the list continues to grow. Some of the oncogenes associated with human tumors are listed below.

abl	– Chronic granulocytic (myelocytic) leukemia
sis	– Osteosarcoma, megakaryoblastic leukemia
L-myc	– Lung, lymphoma, colon, stomach, kidney, prostate, breast
N-myc	– Neuroblastoma
myb	– Teratocarcinoma, melanoma, breast
erb B	– Salivary gland, breast
H ras	– Bladder, breast, colon, rectum, lymphoma, thyroid
B lym	– Burkitt's lymphoma
K ras	– Lung, ovary, stomach, pancreas, colon
N ras	– Acute myelogenous leukemia, neuroblastoma
fes	– Lung, leukemia
dbl	– B-cell lymphoma
egf	– Glioma
raf	– Stomach

hst   – Stomach
akt-1   – Stomach
ros-1   – Glioblastoma
int-2   – Breast
neu   – Breast

The products of some of the oncogenes have been identified and include:

growth factors (e.g. c-sis encodes for platelet derived growth factor)

growth factor receptors (e.g. c-erb-B encodes for epidermal growth factor receptor, c-ros for insulin receptor)

DNA binding proteins (e.g. ras encodes for GTP binding protein)

Protein kinases (e.g. for tyrosine kinase)

Several mechanisms have been identified for the change of a proto-oncogene to an oncogene. These include:

Aberration in gene sequence, including single base pair mutations to deletions or translocations (ras genes are activated as a result of a single base pair mutation at codon 12, 13, or 61).

Aberrant protein product produced as a result of truncated mRNA (c-erb-B and c-erb-B2).

Increase in the levels of mRNA resulting from aberrant gene control, loss of inhibitory or regulatory proteins, gene duplication or amplifications (c-erb-B shown to be amplified in salivary gland adenocarcinoma; c-myc expressed in constitutively high levels in Burkitt's lymphoma).

Inappropriate expression of a gene in a particular cell in a particular stage of differentiation.

Hybrid mRNA resulting from translocation (c-abl and bcr in the 9-22 chromosome translocation in chronic myelogenous leukemia; the bcr-abl protein has phosphotyrosine kinase activity lacking in the normal abl protein).

In African Burkitt's lymphoma an 8-14 chromosomal translocation is seen in 75% of cases. This puts the cmyc gene next to the immunoglobulin areas leading to uncontrolled B-cell proliferation.

There are several important concepts about oncogenes:

a. Proto-oncogenes are likely to be targets of carcinogens and oncogene mutation is likely to be an early step in carcinogenesis.

b. The activation of more than one oncogene may be necessary for development of some cancers.

Oncogenes have been identified in 20–30% of human tumor specimens. Their presence has been correlated in some cancers with prognosis (e.g. those women with the c-erb-B2 oncogene in their breast cancer have a worse prognosis).

In the future, the identification of oncogenes may be important in designing therapy e.g. those neuroblastomas with N-myc amplification need more aggressive therapy. Also, oncogene analysis may help design therapy for different histologic tumors (e.g. an undifferentiated cancer from the liver with a specific oncogene pattern may be more effectively treated with a regimen known to be effective in tumors with that oncogene pattern arising in the lung).

In addition, by knowing the oncogene products, specific antidotes may be developed. We all may be subjected to genetic analysis to see what cancers our genomes predict we may be susceptible to. Knowing this, more targeted prevention and screening programs could be developed.

If only 30% of human cancers are known to have oncogenes now, what about the rest? Do our current technical skills just limit their identification? The answer to this likely is no, and that perhaps there is at least another mechanism. Oncogenes have been shown to stimulate growth. Another class of genes has been shown to retard growth and loss of them may allow for growth out of control. Recently, such genes, called antioncogenes, have been discovered.

There is a rare childhood tumor called retinoblastoma. It can be inherited in an autosomal dominant fashion, and when the inheritance occurs, it has been found to be a loss of part of chromosome 13. On this segment lost, a gene called the Rb gene has been identified, and loss of this is associated with development of retinoblastomas. The ingenious search for this discovery is detailed by Weinberg in *Scientific American* (Sept. 1988, p. 44). Weinberg states that it may in fact be more likely to knock out genes by "crude genetic blows than to hyperactivate it by suble mutational therapy." This type of loss of an antioncogene is seen in Wilms' tumor also. Many other tumors (e.g. small cell carcinoma of the lung) are associated with a non-random loss of part of a chromosome, and perhaps

the loss of anti-oncogenes is a more common phenomenon
activation.

DIFFERENTIATION AND CANCER

A cancer is made up of cells derived from normal tissues; the crucial
difference is lack of normal differentiation. The target cell in tissues for
carcinogenic agents is often (if not always) a committed, but not yet fully
differentiated stem cell or a cell that has the capacity to divide when
further stimulated by mitogenic agents.

Cancer cells are cells that have not achieved a fully differentiated state.
They are blocked at some earlier stage of maturation. Although they may
exhibit some of the characteristics of normal differentiated cells, they
maintain the capacity to divide that most normal differentiated cells lose
as they mature. The growth of tumors may retain dependency on host
factors, at least during some phases of their lifespans, e.g., dependency
on estrogens of some breast tumors, or they may make their own factors,
i.e., the autocrine hypothesis. The microenvironment in which malignant
cells grow is involved in the maintenance of the malignant state. For
example, teratocarcinoma cells, when placed in a normal embryonic environment, differentiate into normal tissues, but when inoculated into
adult liver, kidney, or skin, produce malignant tumors.

The blocked differentiation of cancer cells is not totally irreversible.
Some types of cancer cells can be induced to differentiate to a more mature, less malignant state by exposure to various growth factors or drugs.
Many of the agents that induce differentiation and reduce malignancy of
cultured cells *in vitro* do not appear to stop malignant cell growth *in vivo*.
This may be due to pharmacological problems (e.g., poor absorption of
the agent into the bloodstream, low penetration into tissues, rapid metabolism, or rapid excretion of the agent). In addition, the continual presence of the inducer might be required until the cells are past a critical
stage of differentiation. There is also the possibility that the adult stroma
in which the cancer cells arise does not usually favor differentiation of
these cells. At any rate, the possibility that the malignant state of certain
types of cancer cells is potentially reversible holds out the hope that therapies aimed at stimulating differentiation are possible.

ANAPLASIA

One of the major hallmarks of cancer is anaplasia (derived from the Greek plasia—form, ana—prior to), meaning the cells look young, disorganized, and often "angry." The cancer cells have failed to differentiate to their adult state, and in so doing, they may possess antigens not usually expressed in the adult cell (e.g. carcinoembryonic antigen (CEA) or alphafetoprotein (AFP).

Other types of "plasias" include:

Dysplasia—Growth without form, e.g. dysplasia (or disorganization) of the cervical mucosa that occurs prior to cervical cancer or bronchial dysplasia preceding lung cancer.

Hyperplasia—Increased cellularity. Hyperplasia (especially if there are "atypical" features) may precede breast or endometrial cancer.

Metaplasia—Change of one type of adult epithelium for another e.g. in Barrett's esophagus change of the squamous epithelium to glandular epithelium precedes the development of adenocarcinomas in that region.

TUMOR GROWTH

Tumors develop from single cells. As the cells grow, genetic instability occurs and with progression, multiple clones may be seen. This is illustrated in Figure 3.1.

The tumor begins from a single cell and may evolve to be a tumor mass with multiple clones with different chromosomal numbers as seen here and with different properties.

This can explain why differences in sensitivity to cancer therapies exist in cells even within the same tumor, e.g. some may be sensitive and some resistant to the same chemotherapeutic agent. Therapy may even select for the evolution of more resistant clones.

This heterogeneity may also explain why some serological "tumor markers" may not always reflect the status of the tumor.

KINETICS

In the past, the growth of tumors was believed to follow the principles of Gompertzian growth, i.e., an S-shaped curve with decremental growth at

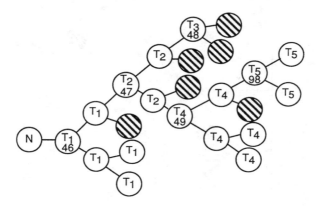

Figure 3.1. *Tumor Cell Heterogeneity.* As tumors progress, more aneuploidy develops, some cells die, and others become resistant to therapies or take on properties that make them more likely to disseminate.

larger sizes. However, Norton and Simon have challenged the Gompertzian model of tumor growth. Their model says that there is a lag phase as the *beginning* of tumor growth (as well as a slowdown with large numbers of tumor cells). Their model predicts that the largest doses of therapy should be given when there are few cells left (i.e., "crescendo therapy").

Cancer cells need a source of nutrients and oxygen to sustain growth. After reaching a certain size, a substance called "tumor angiogenesis factor" is elaborated, which stimulates the growth of capillaries into the tumor. Tumors will not grow larger than 3–4 mm unless vascularization occurs.

A typical growth curve for a tumor is shown in Figure 3.2.

Of note, it takes 10^9 cells to first have a detectable tumor (e.g. a 1 cm mass seen on CXR or felt on rectal exam). This represents three-quarters of the natural history of a tumor. The lethal tumor burden is usually somewhere between 10^{12}-10^{13} cells.

The period from the time of neoplastic transformation until a clinical tumor is seen is called the latent period. If we could diagnose tumors during this preclinical period, there would be a much greater likelihood

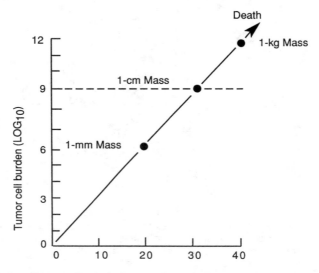

Figure 3.2. *Tumor Growth Curve.* Tumors begin from single cells. With present technology, they cannot be detected until 10^9 cells are present.

of "cure." Some cancers (e.g. cervical cancer) can be diagnosed before they are seen with the naked eye (e.g. by "Pap" smears). Others may use markers e.g. elevation of HCG in a choriocarcinoma arising out of pregnancy.

One important concept about tumor growth is the concept of doubling time. This is the time it takes a measurable tumor to double in size and represents cell gain and cell loss. Tumors with faster doubling times are more likely to respond to chemotherapy because chemotherapy is more likely to affect dividing cells. However, some tumors with slower doubling times may still respond quite well since they may have rapid turnover of cells with a lot of cell death, causing a slower increase in size.

Doubling time tends to increase as tumors enlarge. This slowdown of growth usually makes these larger tumors more refractory to chemotherapy. It is likely that most smaller tumors are growing faster and are more likely to respond.

BRIEF REVIEW OF TUMOR BIOLOGY

Because of the loss of contact inhibition of movement and mitoses, the abnormal motility, the increased tissue pressure of the expanding mass, the decreased cell-to-cell cohesion, and the lack of growth of regulatory intercellular communications, tumor cells expand locally and invade local tissues. Furthermore, secreted enzymes like hyaluronidase may facilitate invasion. Microscopic invasion is often far removed from the gross borders of a cancer; hence the use of wide excisions in surgery.

METASTASES

If cancers remain localized to the site of origin, local excision or local radiotherapy may be curative. Cancers have differing tendencies to disseminate from the primary site, and when dealing with a specific neoplasm, the known behavior of that type of cancer should be taken into account when deciding upon therapy.

Cancer cells may invade vessels or lymphatics. Tumor cells are less adhesive to other cells, and single cells or clumps may break off to be spread to distant sites. Many more cells are shed than the ones that produce metastases ($>1000 \times$). The bloodstream is an adverse environment, and most cells die. The viability of detached neoplastic cells is probably more easily preserved in the lymphatic channels. Cells are more likely to break off at the periphery of a growth where the growth rate and viability of the cells are greatest.

Circulating tumor cells are attacked by N-K cells, PMNs, and mononuclear cells. Attachment to platelets or fibrin clots may protect from immune destruction and facilitate implantation.

Cells adhere to the vessel walls with the help of fibrin strands probably present at "gaps" in endothelial walls where endothelial renewal is occurring or through the help of platelets adhered to their surfaces. It is likely that cells adhere to receptors like those for laminin and fibronectin. The cells that adhere are a select few and may differ from the primary tumor in substantial aspects. Large clumps of tumor cells may wedge in small capillaries. The clotting system is often abnormal in cancer, e.g., low grade DIC. Heparin and Coumadin have been shown to decrease experimental metastases. Also, platelets must be very important. Substances which inhibit platelet adhesion decrease metastases in experimental models. Many trials are in progress utilizing the anticoagulant drugs to astases in man. Other trials are trying to increase the effec- he attacking cells like N-K cells.

therent, diapedesis into tissue space (or bursting after intra- growth) occurs. Tumor angiogenesis again begins, and the secondary growth behaves in somewhat the same fashion as the early primary growth. Metastatic deposits may lie dormant for years also.

It is not known why metastases go to certain organs as shown in Table 3.1. In part, it is related to blood flow, but also there may be true organotropism for certain sites. The metastatic process is probably not random. It involves selection of cells with certain properties. Metastatic cells may be *very* different from the primary in numerous characteristics because of this selective process.

Cancer cells may enter lymphatics either directly or through the venous system. Local nodes are the first line of defense for many cancers,

Table 3.1
Most Frequent Sites of Metastasis from Some Human Carcinomas

Primary Tumor	Most Frequent Sites of Metastasis
Breast	Axillary lymph nodes, opposite breast, lung, pleura, liver, bone, brain, adrenal, spleen, and ovary
Colon	Regional lymph nodes, liver, lung, by direct extension to urinary bladder or stomach
Kidney	Lung, liver, and bone
Lung	Regional lymph nodes, pleura, diaphragm (by direct extension) liver, bone, brain, kidney, adrenal, thyroid, and spleen
Ovary	Peritoneum, regional lymph nodes
Prostate	Bones of spine and pelvis, regional lymph nodes
Stomach	Regional lymph nodes, liver, lung, and bone
Testis	Regional lymph nodes, lung, and liver
Urinary bladder	By direct extension to rectum, colon, prostate, ureter, vagina, bone; regional lymph nodes; bone; lung; peritoneum; pleura; liver; and brain
Uterine endometrium	Regional lymph nodes, lung, liver, and ovary

especially epithelial. Why some tumors spread by lymphatics and others by veins is unknown. Some tumors like ovarian cancer have tropism for serosal surfaces.

Some of the author's rules about metastases:

1. Breast cancer and melanoma can do anything!

2. Unknown primary is often an unusual metastatic pattern for its tumor of origin.

3. Unknown primary cancer in a woman is breast cancer until proven otherwise.

4. Prostate cancer hardly ever produces nodules in the lungs or brain. (It does sometime, though!)

5. Get a good biopsy; talk personally to the pathologist. Remember electron microscopy, estrogen receptors, immunohistochemistry, epidemiology, and special stains often help with the diagnosis.

IMPORTANT POINTS FOR THE HOUSE OFFICER

1. It is likely that discoveries arising from the biology of cancer will lead to new therapies or new strategies for prevention.

2. Oncogenes and anti-oncogenes seem very promising for understanding the basic mechanisms of carcinogenesis. For example, the presence of oncogenes may define susceptibility; the pattern of oncogenes may define therapy, and oncogene products or anti-oncogene (suppressor) products may be very useful in the treatment of cancer.

3. To understand cancer and its therapies one must understand cell kinetics. Tumor cell heterogeneity which occurs as neoplasms progress may explain refractiveness to therapy.

4. Understanding and stopping the metastatic process may provide useful therapies.

5. Eliminating promoters or adding anti-promoters may delay or eliminate cancers. During this phase of carcinogenesis, irreversible changes may not yet have occurred, and "differentiation" back to the normal phenotype may occur.

Chapter 4

Primary Prevention of Cancer

CAUSES OF CANCER

Let us examine what is said to "cause" cancer. The list in Table 4.1 comes from the work of Doll and Peto (*JNCI* 66(6):1191–1308, 1981).

Doll and Peto have surveyed the world's literature to develop this list, which as you see contains a "best estimate" and a range. Some cancers are clearly multifactorial, and the exact roles of certain factors like diet and infection are subject to much debate.

Table 4.1
Causes of Cancer Mortality

Factor or Class of Factors	Percent of All Cancer Deaths	
	Best Estimate	*Range of Acceptable Estimates*
Tobacco	30%	25–40%
Alcohol	3%	2–4%
Diet	35%	10–70%
Reproductive and sexual behavior	7%	1–13%
Occupation	4%	2–8%
Pollution	2%	1–5%
Industrial products	1%	1–2%
Medicines and medical procedures	1%	0.5–3%
Geophysical factors	3%	2–4%

One very important aspect of cancer causation that this list clearly illustrates is how much *personal behaviors* (like smoking or diet) are responsible for cancer. It is also becoming more clear that these factors can be much more devastating acting on a "receptive" genome.

TYPES OF PREVENTION

There are three types of prevention: primary, secondary, and tertiary.

Primary prevention involves eliminating the cause for the cancer before it begins. Theoretically, this is the best and probably most cost-effective way to control cancer. Currently, there are many factors which make primary prevention difficult to apply, e.g. changing behavior even when the carcinogen is known (smoking) or pinpointing the specific dietary factors associated with cancer.

There are three levels of primary prevention. They can simply be stated as follows.

The government does everything, the individual nothing.

The government does something, the individual something.

The individual does everything.

The government gets its data for possible cancer causation mainly from three sources: (1) human epidemiological studies; (2) animal studies (which are often long and costly); and (3) short-term *in vitro* assays, especially the Ames assay which tests chemicals to see if they are mutagens. These *in vitro* assays are quick and relatively cheap. If a chemical is a mutagen in the Ames test, animal studies are then performed.

The government's regulatory agencies include:

The Environmental Protection Agency (EPA), which has broad responsibilities, including monitoring and regulating ambient air and water pollution, solid wastes, noise, pesticides, and radiation hazards.

The Occupational Safety and Health Administration (OSHA) (in the Department of Labor), which regulates hazards in the workplace. OSHA cannot ban the production or use of hazardous chemicals, but can require that workers be protected from exposure to them.

The Consumer Product Safety Commission (CPSC) regulates the composition of consumer products and the uses for which they can be recommended to protect the health and well-being of the user. (However, tobacco and tobacco products are specifically excluded from CPSC's authority.)

The Nuclear Regulatory Commission (NRC) regulates the use of nuclear materials.

The Food and Drug Administration (FDA) protects human health from unsafe foods or additives, and drugs, cosmetics and medical devices. A special feature of the food law is its regulation of additives found to cause cancer by the "Delaney Clause i.e. the FDA may ban the use of a food additive "if it is found to induce cancer when ingested by man or animal, or if it is found, after tests which are appropriate for the evaluation of the safety of food additives, to induce cancer in man or animal. . . ."

There also are governmental research organizations involved with identifying carcinogens. These include the National Cancer Institute (NCI), the National Institute of Environmental Health Services, and the National Institute of Occupational Health and Safety.

These agencies work in the first two levels of prevention. In the first level, where the government does everything, an agency may regulate a product out of existence, e.g., red dye #2. The second level is where there is a great deal of controversy. The government identifies a product as a potential carcinogen, but other factors (e.g., economic, political, etc.) are also important. An example is aflatoxin, which is a very potent carcinogen. Aflatoxin adheres to corn, but corn is an extremely important foodstuff. To resolve the dilemma, the government sets levels that are acceptable for ingestion, carefully weighing the risk of cancer and benefits of corn as a food.

A recent example of the risk-benefit analysis is the saccharin story. By the Delaney Clause, the government has a right to ban saccharin, and the FDA moved to implement a ban when it was found to be carcinogenic in rats. However, protest letters to Congress because of the presumed "benefits" of saccharin caused them to defeat the FDA sponsored bill, and saccharin remains on the market.

Secondary prevention is discovery of the cancer at an early stage, amenable to "curative" therapy. This is also called screening, and will be the subject of Chapter 5.

Tertiary prevention is the prevention of cancer in patients who have already experienced one cancer. Such patients (e.g., smokers "cured" of one head and neck cancer) will be at very great risk to develop another cancer (if they continue to smoke). Tertiary prevention includes precepts of both primary and secondary prevention and won't be discussed per se in this chapter.

PERSPECTIVE

When one reads the popular press, one gets the impression that "everything causes cancer." It is true that we live in an environment loaded with known carcinogens, but to effectively apply the principles of primary prevention, one must put into perspective the concept of relative risk. There are many factors that lead to confusion about relative risk. What people perceive as risks has a very large emotional component. The consumer has a difficult time sorting out risks, especially when risks are very low.

Bruce Ames, who developed the Ames test for evaluation of mutagenicity, has tried to help quantify risk by developing a ranking of carcinogens. He calls this the "HERP (Human Exposure Rodent Potency) Index" (*Science* 236:271–280, 1987), and it compares the human exposure to a dose in rodents known to produce a certain number of tumors. There is a great deal of controversy about this index, but it is an attempt to quantify risk. To make the biggest gains, we should focus our efforts on those things that produce the biggest risks.

In any attempt to quantitate risks, it is clear that the biggest risks are our personal habits, and these should be subject to change, although behavioral change can be exceedingly difficult to bring about.

SOME SPECIFIC STRATEGIES FOR PRIMARY PREVENTION

Smoking

Smoking is known to be associated with 30% of cancer deaths, and if one counts deaths from other causes associated with smoking, there are 390,000 deaths per year in the U.S. Former Surgeon General Koop calls smoking "the chief single avoidable cause of death in our society and the most important public health issue of our time."

There is no question that all forms of smoking are associated with cancer. The cancer risk increases with intensity of the habit, duration, and the amount of tar in cigarettes. Stopping smoking decreases the risk, but it is not clear whether the risk declines to that of nonsmokers.

The percentage of smokers, especially among males, is declining in the U.S., but worldwide, especially in the less developed countries, smoking is becoming more prevalent. In the U.S., the percentage of males who smoke has declined from 52.4% of those over 20 in 1965 to 33.2% in 1985. In women, the rates were 34.1% in 1965 and 27.9% in 1985.

There is also convincing data that "passive" smoking or exposure to second-hand smoke increases cancer risk in non-smokers. The evidence is detailed in a 1986 report by the Surgeon General and is available by calling 1-800-4-CANCER.

How can the house officer affect smoking habits? Here are some of the suggestions the author has found useful:

A. The best way to decrease smoking is to get people never to start. Whenever you take a history, ask about smoking and compliment patients, especially younger ones, when they say they don't smoke. Reinforce their behavior, even though the media may be sending messages that smoking is sophisticated, sexy, "cool," associated with fun and an active lifestyle. There exist many "teachable" moments for families, e.g. when a loved one is diagnosied with a smoking related condition. Utilize these "moments" to try to influence family members to get across the message *not* to smoke.

B. For your patients who do smoke, I would suggest the method of Judy Okene. This is described in the *Archives of Internal Medicine* (148:1039–1045, 1988).

First, you should ask your patients if they smoke, and if so, how much and how long. A simple message that "you should quit for health reasons" delivered by a physician *does* have an impact, and every one of your patients who smokes should be viewed as a candidate for cessation.

Next, you should assist the patients in implementing a plan. Okene uses the following model.

1. Get the details of the patients' smoking history. (How much? When started? Prior attempts at quitting?)

2. Advise cessation. Be positive—let it be known you believe in your patient's ability to stop. Positive outcomes are correlated with expectations of success by both the patient and you.

3. Personalize the risks of smoking and benefits of quitting, but don't use fear tactics. State objectively and honestly the health risks of smoking. Is there a family history of smoking related disease? Are there symptoms (cough, decreased exercise tolerance, etc)? Are there signs on physical exam (ronchi, wheezes, nicotine stained fingers or teeth, wrinkles, smoker's breath, etc.)? Some physicians have a spirometer or a carbon monoxide meter in their office to demonstrate the harmful effects objectively.

4. Assess motivation. Are they ready to quit? If not, to cut down? What are the reasons? (The more reasons the greater the chance of success.) Help them find reasons, e.g., disease states to avoid.

5. Assess past experiences. 40–60% of smokers have quit before. It often takes multiple attempts to quit. What were the pitfalls or problems.? How can they be avoided this time?

6. Discuss problems. Make them aware of nicotine withdrawal symptoms, and how to cope with them. Discuss times that may lead to temptation.

7. Discuss resources. (Here are some aids available for free.)

	Available From
How to Quit Cigarettes	American Cancer Society
I Quit Kit	American Cancer Society
Freedom From Smoking in 20 Days	American Lung Assn.
A Lifetime of Freedom From Smoking	American Lung Assn.
Me Quit Smoking? How?	American Lung Assn.
How to Stop Smoking	American Heart Assn.
Smoker's Self-Testing Kit	U.S. Dept. of Health & Human Services, Office on Smoking and Health, Park Bldg 1-58, Rockville, MD 20857

Clearing the Air   National Cancer Institute
                                Bethesda, MD 20205

8. There is no "right way" to stop. Different ways work for different people. Some suggest using aversive techniques like rapid smoking (e.g. keep on inhaling rapidly to the point of feeling sick), or behavioral modification (e.g. rating "value" of each cigarette—dropping out those of least value or only smoking in certain places at certain times).

9. Negotiate a plan for change. If they are not ready to "cold turkey," plan for a cutdown or switch to a lower tar brand. Write out the plan, set a date and sign it together.

10. Arrange a follow-up (see below)

Here is a sample intervention:

Doctor: "Smoking is harmful to your health. In many cases, the harmful effects of smoking can be reversed. As your doctor, I must advise you to stop smoking because . . . (personalize to patient)."

Have you thought about stopping?

What reasons would you have for stopping?

Have you ever actually stopped smoking?

Yes	*No*
• When was the last time?	• Have you every made any other changes in your smoking? What?
• How did you stop?	
• Any problems?	
• How long did the problem last?	• When? Any problems?
• What helped you?	
• How did you feel?	

Would you like to stop smoking?

Do you think you could stop smoking?

What would be possible problems associated with stopping?

What could help you?

Would you be willing to develop a plan to stop smoking?

Yes	*No*

- Write Plan for Change with patient (see below)
- Give booklet on tips for stopping smoking (see above)
- Review factors that may interfere with plan.
- Request return visit in 1–2 weeks (or phone contact if visit impossible) to check progress.

- Would you be willing to cut down on your smoking?
- If yes, write Plan for Change (tapering) with patient.
- Give booklet on tips for stopping smoking.
- Review factors that may interfere with plan.
- Request return visit in 1–2 weeks (or phone contact if visit impossible) to check progress.

Okene teaches physicians to have patients sign the following plan for change.

PLAN FOR CHANGE

I, _____ , hereby promise to myself that I will stop smoking cigarettes on _____ .

My reasons for stopping are:

_____
_____
_____
_____

Steps I will take to achieve stopping are:

_____
_____
_____
_____

Date _____   Signed _____

She also distributes these "comebacks" to frequently asked questions.

1. P: I am under a lot of stress, and smoking relaxes me.

    A: Your body has become accustomed to nicotine, so you naturally feel more relaxed when you get the nicotine you have come to depend on. But nicotine is actually a stimulant that temporarily raises heart rate, blood pressure, and adrenaline level. After a few weeks of not smoking, most ex-smokers feel less nervous.

2. P: Smoking stimulates me and helps me to be more effective in my work.

    A: Difficulty in concentrating can be a symptom of nicotine withdrawal, but it is a short-term effect. Over time, the body and brain function more efficiently when you don't smoke, because carbon monoxide from cigarettes is displaced by oxygen in the bloodstream.

3. P: I have already cut down to a safe level.

    A: Cutting down is a good first step toward quitting. But smoking at any level increases the risk of illness. And some smokers who cut back inhale more often and more deeply, thus maintaining nicotine dependence. It is best to quit smoking completely.

4. P: I only smoke safe, low-tar/low-nicotine cigarettes.

    A: Low-tar cigarettes still contain harmful substances. Many smokers inhale more often or more deeply and thus maintain their nicotine levels. Carbon monoxide intake often increases with a switch to low-tar cigarettes.

5. P: I don't have the willpower to give up smoking.

    A: It can be hard for some people to give up smoking but for others it is much easier than they expect. More than 3 million Americans quit every year. It may take more than one attempt for you to succeed, and you may need to try different methods of quitting. I will give you all the support I can.

The final part of the plan is follow-up. This is very important. Patients need a great deal of help to quit this very addictive habit. In follow-up sessions, if they have quit, make sure to congratulate them, and to assess their problem areas (e.g., weight gain, irritability, etc.). If they haven't been able to quit, review the plan, and the difficulties they had and problem-solve with them to get a successful plan.

A recent addition to the armamentarium to help patients stop is nicotine gum (Nicorette®). Here are the instructions that should be given to patients:

1. Begin use of Nicorette® only when you have *completely* stopped the use of cigarettes.

2. Follow instructions and guidelines included with the Nicorette® prescription.

3. Keep your Nicorette® with you at all times where you usually keep your cigarettes. Remember, this is a prescription drug. Do not let anyone else use your Nicorette®. Keep it out of reach of children. Do not take if pregnant or breast feeding.

4. When you feel you need a cigarette put one piece of gum in your mouth.

5. Chew the gum very slowly until you feel a slight tingling in your mouth or taste the gum (usually occurs after about 15 chews). At this time stop chewing and park the gum between your cheek and teeth until the tingling or taste stops. Begin to chew slowly again until the tingling or taste reappears. At this time, again park the gum between your teeth and cheek (alternate cheeks). This process of chewing and parking the gum is similar to puffing on a cigarette and putting it down or holding it until your ready to take another drag. Chewing slowly is necessary to allow the nicotine in the gum to be absorbed gradually by your body. After about 30 minutes, all of the nicotine will be absorbed.

6. Most people find 10–15 pieces/day of Nicorette® are enough to control their urge to smoke. However, use as many as are necessary the first few days after you stop smoking, but it is recommended that you do not use more than 30 pieces a day. Side effects may be caused by using the gum incorrectly or too fast. Here is a list of these side effects: lightheadedness, nausea/vomiting, throat and mouth irritation, hiccups, stomach upset, mouth ulcers, jaw muscle ache, headaches, heart palpitations, and more than usual amount of saliva in the mouth. Report any symptoms.

Even by providing advice, follow-up, and if necessary, the use of gum, "quit" rates are only about 15–20%, but even this will make a significant impact on future heath. The above is the advice for you to try to help your patients on your own. There are many resources available in hospitals and communities. You should contact the patient education program of your hospital to find out about these, as well as your local chapters of the American Cancer Society, the American Heart Association and/or the American Lung Association. You also can contact the Cancer Information Service at 1-800-4-CANCER to find out places to refer your patients.

C. In addition to trying to change smoking behavior in individuals, physicians should act on a community and societal level. Become volunteers in your local ACS. Be vocal and share your expertise with school boards, local business groups and local government. Speak out about your hospital going "smoke free." Become aware of national and state laws about health promotion and support these, especially with letters and calls to legislators.

Join the American Medical Association, or the American Academy of Family Physicians (which has recently developed an excellent smoking cessation kit), Doctors Ought to Care (DOC) or the American College of Physicians. All these have joined the efforts to decrease smoking.

D. Tobacco in the form of cigarettes is most strongly associated with cancer, but you should also be aware that smoking pipes and/or cigars is also associated. The use of "smokeless" tobacco is associated with cancer of the mouth, and should be emphatically discouraged.

Dietary Interventions

The data on diet and cancer are controversial, and in some cases associations are very "soft." Despite this, recommendations have been made by many national bodies and they seem to be "reasonable" suggestions for people to live by. Most of the suggestions on diet and cancer also would be the same for heart disease, and adoption of a healthier diet by U.S. citizens seems prudent.

The rules for diet in some ways are similar now to what they have always been. Simply stated, one should:

1. Eat as wide a variety of food as possible, and

2. Everything in moderation. (Mark Twain is said to have added to this "including moderation.")

To summarize the recommendations of the National Academy of Sciences (1989), the Surgeon General (1988), the NCI (1986), and the ACS (1984):

1. *Avoid:*
   • Obesity—excess caloric intake

2. *Decrease/Moderate Intake of:*
   • Fat—to no more than 30% of calories

- Alcohol—to maximum of 2 drinks/day or less (none if driving!)
- Salt-cured, nitrate-cured, smoked, and pickled foods

3. *Increase Intake of Foods Containing*
   - Fiber—cereal grains, fruits and vegetables
   - Beta-Carotene—fruits and vegetables
   - Vitamin C—fruits and vegetables

Let me review each of these briefly with some suggestions for the house officer.

1. Obesity. In the U.S., the intake of too many calories is far too prevalent. Obesity is associated with breast, endometrial, and gallbladder cancer. Much has been written about "how to" lose weight, but simply put, one must decrease calorie intake, increase energy output, or a combination of both.

2. Fat. We also take in too many calories from fat. The strongest association with fat intake appears to be with cancer of the colon, but it also has been associated with cancer of the pancreas. The link with breast, endometrial, ovarian, and prostate cancer is less clear. By decreasing fat, one also decreases calories and helps lower cholesterol. The recommendation for the ratio of saturated to unsaturated fat in the diet is not clear. Some studies and models show that unsaturated fat may be more of a risk for cancer, but this certainly isn't entirely clear. I feel we should limit total fat and balance saturated and unsaturated fat.

Doctors are not taught what is in "food." We have difficulty telling our patients what to eat because most of us don't know food composition. I have two strategies:

A. Refer patients to the dieticians.

B. Recommend Jane Brody's *Nutrition Book* (Bantam Books, 1982, $8.95). Here are some of her suggestions for decreasing fat:

   (1) Decrease meat intake—smaller servings, "meatless" meals, substitute by using poultry (cut off skin) or fish.

   (2) Choose lean meats—avoid well-marbled meats, trim off fat, buy "lean beef."

   (3) Boil or roast rather than fry.

   (4) Skim off the fat from stew or soups.

(5) Switch to low fat milk. Use milk in coffee; restrict intake of hard and processed cheeses.

(6) Use yogurt in place of sour cream.

(7) Use margarine or polyunsaturated vegetable oils. The less hard the margarine, the less saturated it will be.

3. Alcohol will be discussed below.

4. Avoid salt cured, nitrate cured, smoked, and pickled food. Remember, everything in moderation.

5. Fiber. What fiber does for cancer is by no means clear, but ads on television make it seem like the "cureall." Fiber does help bowel regularity, and may lower cholesterol. Eating more fiber probably makes us eat less fat and calories. If any type does, the fiber most likely to decrease cancer is not from grain, but from fruits and vegetables. The latter, especially cruciferous vegetables (broccoli, cauliflower, Brussels sprouts, kale, cabbage), may contain "anti-carcinogens."

6. Carotene/Vitamin C. These may be protectors against cancer. Much data says the best place to get these is probably from food, not taking an extra pill to compensate for a poor diet. Again, fruits and vegetables may be key. There are many ongoing studies investigating the role of these vitamins given as supplements and the incidence of cancer. Are they chemoprevention agents? At this point, we do not know.

7. Although not mentioned, some scientists view protein as a possible culprit. Like fat and calories, we in the U.S. eat levels of protein far above the Recommended Dietary Allowances (RDA). Protein stimulates hormones which may in turn be growth factors for cancers. High protein intake is related to the development of osteoporosis, which is a cause of major morbidity in the U.S.

Remember also that diet must be individualized to meet any specific physiologic requirements a person has. One other aspect of diet worth mentioning for the house officer is that this is a very "ripe" area for faddism and quackery. Remember the rules that nothing is safe until proven to be safe and nothing is efficacious until proven to be.

Many unsubstantiated claims are made about diet and cancer. There is no "anti-cancer diet," but the sound practices outlined above are the current best way to avoid cancer. The subject of food faddism is reviewed by Dr. Victor Herbert in *Nutrition and Cancer* (6:96, 1984).

Alcohol

Alcohol accounts for 3% of cancer. Alcohol plus tobacco are strongly synergistic.

The house officer should recognize the early signs of alcohol abuse. We have found the CAGE screen (with positive answers to at least two of the four questions) to be useful. The questions are:

1. Have you ever felt you ought to *Cut* down on drinking?
2. Have people *Annoyed* you by criticizing your drinking?
3. Have you ever felt bad or *Guilty* about your drinking?
4. Have you have had a drink first thing in the morning to steady your nerves or get rid of a hangover (*Eyeopener*)?

Early referral to an alcohol counseling service can be lifesaving.

Radiation

From Doll and Peto's data, radiation is said to account for 1% of cancer. We are all exposed to natural background radiation, but the largest other source of radiation to the population is through medical x-rays. You as the gatekeeper can control to a certain extent the number of x-rays your patients get. Always ask, is it necessary? What will I learn? Could the patient be pregnant? As a consumer, you should ask your dentist if you really need those "bite wing" x-rays. These are only a few of the questions you might ask. Be careful with your exposure to radiation.

Much has been written lately about exposure to radon. Radon is a gas produced by the breakdown of radium or its parent element uranium. "Natural" pockets of radon have been found. All states have detectable levels, but higher levels have been found in Pennsylvania, Colorado, New Jersey, Florida, and New Hampshire. The Environmental Protection Agency has found that 12% of the homes they assessed contain levels of radon that warrant reduction by the homeowner, but only 1% of homes surveyed have dangerous levels. Radon has been associated especially with lung cancer, and the estimates of deaths per year range from several thousand to over twenty thousand.

Radon present in the rocks and soil is released into the air and groundwater. It may seep in through cracks in basement walls, or be released in bathrooms through the running water from deep wells. The greater levels of insulation spurred on by the energy conservation movement tend to keep radon trapped, especially in basements. Breakdown products of radon in the air may become attached to dust particles or drops of moisture, and when people breath these in, they can irradiate lung tissue.

Your state health department can tell you if you live and practice in an area of high risk. The ACS has special expertise in answering questions about radon.

Screening test measurements which are taken under closed-house conditions in the lowest livable level of a house for from one to five days may be done to estimate levels to which household inhabitants are exposed. If a screening test indicates a problem, long-term and more accurate testing can be done to estimate the annual average exposure, with measurements taken over four seasons in normal living conditions. If the laboratory analysis based on information collected for this test indicates that the level of radon gas is higher than the EPA's recommended limit (four picocuries of radon per liter of air), some contractors have the expertise to be able to reduce the entry of radon gas into your home or to provide for better ventilation of the gas. Also, the EPA offers publications that describe how to reduce the entry of radon into the home.

Ultraviolet Light

There is a rapid rise in those cancers felt due to ultraviolet light exposure (basal cell and squamous cell carcinomas of the skin ard malignant melanoma). Many factors are felt to be contributory, the most important of which seem to be the changes in clothing habits exposing more skin to ultraviolet light damage, the increase in leisure time with associated increase in sun exposure, and the societal value placed on a suntan as a sign of health. Furthermore, depletion of the ozone layer and the production of chlorofluorocarbons, which in the past were present in aerosol sprays, has allowed more ultraviolet radiation to penetrate and this may be associated with this increased rate of malignant melanoma.

People with fair skin are at increased risk for skin cancers. Some specific suggestions to decrease the risk include:

1. Avoid prolonged exposure to U.V. radiation. Since the most intense exposure occurs between 10:00 a.m. and 2:00 p.m., minimize unprotected exposure during this period.

2. Wear sunscreens. SPF means solar protection factor and many sunscreens are available commercially with SPF's of 15 or greater. Apply these frequently (about every 2–3 hours for direct prolonged exposure).

3. Remember that even on cloudy days, U.V. damage can occur. Also, remember that snow and sand reflect the rays and that immersion in water does not block them.

4. Wear protective clothing—shirts with a collar, brimmed hats, etc.

5. Avoid getting a sunburn, especially one which blisters.

A relatively new development in U.V. light exposure is the increasing use of artificial tanning salons and machines. The long-range effects of this type of exposure are not known. U.V. light is made up of U.V-A and U.V.-B, and the latter is what is felt to be most carcinogenic. U.V.-A is the type of exposure produced by the newest artificial tanning machines and it may be less carcinogenic. However, U.V.-A light penetrates deeper into the dermis, and the tan produced doesn't seem as protective or long-lasting as that produced by natural sunlight. Further, animal studies have shown that it can cause skin cancer and premature aging of the skin.

At this time, it is felt there is no way to get a tan indoors or outdoors without damaging the skin and increasing the risk of skin cancer.

Occupation

In 1775, Sir Percival Pott was the first to describe occupational cancer when he made the link between scrotal cancer and chimney sweeps. Doll and Peto say that 4% of cancers are due to occupational exposures.

Table 4.2 has a partial list of those occupations felt to be associated.

The house officer should take a careful occupational and exposure history in each of his or her patients. Alert clinicians have been able to note

Table 4.2
Established Occupational Causes of Cancer

Site of Cancer	Possible carcinogen	Occupation
Bladder	Aromatic amines rubber workers, coal manufacturers	Dye manufacturers, gas
Skin, lung	Arsenic	Copper and cobalt smelters, arsenical pesticide manufacturers, some gold miners
Lung, pleura,	Asbestos	Asbestos miners, asbestos peritoneum textile manufacturers, asbestos insulation workers, certain shipyard workers
Leukemia	Benzene	Workers with glues and varnishes
Lung	Chromium	Manufacturers of chromates from chrome ore, pigment manufacturers
Lung, bone, bone marrow	Ionizing radiations	Uranium and some other miners, luminizers, radiographers
Nasal sinuses	Isopropyl oil	Isopropyl alcohol manufacturers
Larynx, lung	Mustard gas	Poison gas manufacturers
Nasal sinuses, lung	Nickel	Nickel refiners
Skin, scrotum, lung	Polycyclic hydrocarbons, soot, tar, oil	Coal gas manufacturers roofers, asphalters, aluminium refiners
Liver (angiosarcoma)	Vinyl chloride	PVC manufacturers
Nasal sinuses	(Unknown agent)	Hardwood furniture manufacturers, leather workers

many links in the past, and we all should continue to be alert to possible occupational associations.

Medications

America is a drug conscious society. Many cancers are known to be related to drug use, but with the magnitude of agents used in our population, many more cancers may be attributed to drugs in the future. Table 4.3 lists some of the drugs considered to be related to cancer.

Infection

In Doll and Peto's estimates, infection may account for 10% of cancers. There have been many clusters of cancer seen (e.g. Hodgkin's disease), but as yet no definitive infectious agent has been found to explain the clusters.

There is an increased incidence of cancer in some areas of chronic inflammation, e.g. in the sinus tract draining an area of osteomyelitis, in the biliary tree infected by *Clonorchis* or in the tongue with a chancre from syphilis. Also, cancers occur more frequently in lung "scars" which may be due to infection, e.g. a tuberculosis scar.

Viruses are well known and well proven to produce cancer in other species. To date, only two definitive cancer causing viruses have been identified—the HTLV-I and II viruses, members of the oncornavirus family. HTLV-I causes a T cell lymphoma, or acute T cell oncornaleukemia. The virus is found endemically in areas of southern Japan and in the Caribbean. Antibodies to the virus and copies of the genome are seen in patients with these unusual T cell tumors. Interestingly, 50% of their family members also have antibodies to the virus and 12% of the blood donors from these endemic areas also possess antibodies. The meaning of these latter two facts is as yet unknown.

HTLV-II causes an unusual type of hairy cell leukemia. The virus was identified in a patient with this disease who was an Aleutian from Alaska.

Other viruses have also been implicated, but their exact roles are not entirely clear. The most commonly associated viruses include: Epstein-

Table 4.3
Medications and Cancer

Drug	Use	Related Cancer
Radioisotopes		
Phosphorus ^{32}P	Polycythermia vera	Leukemia
Radium	Tuberculosis (no longer used)	Osteosarcoma, nasal sinus cancer
Thoratrast	Diagnostic radiology (no longer used)	Angiosarcoma of liver
Immunosuppressive drugs		
Antilymphocyte serum	Transplants	Lymphoma
Antimetabolites	Cancer therapy	Sarcoma, liver, skin
Cytotoxic drugs		
Alkylating agents-melphalan, cytoxan	Cancer therapy	Leukemia, bladder
Estrogens		
Prenatal	Morning sickness	Clear cell vaginal cancer in offspring
Postnatal	Multiple use	Endometrial cancer, breast cancer in women who used DES during pregnancy ? liver cancer
Androgens		
Anabolic steroids	Anaplastic anemia, body building	Liver cancer
Other drugs		
Arsenic	Skin tonics	Skin cancer
Phenacetin	Pain	Renal pelvis
Coal tar ointments	Psoriasis	Skin cancer
Dilantin	Seizures	Lymphoma (rare)
Chloramphenicol	Infections	Leukemia (rare)

Barr virus, herpes simplex II, human papilloma virus, and hepatitis B virus.

Epstein-Barr virus has been strongly associated with the African type of Burkitt's lymphoma. Patients with this have high antibody titers, and pieces of viral genome have been found in the tumor DNA. Furthermore, EBV has been shown to transform lymphocytes both in culture and in subhuman primates. However, not all patients infected with EBV get Burkitt's, and in other parts of the world, EBV has not been found to be associated. In Africa, there seems also to be an association with malaria, which may be acting as a promoter. It is unlikely that EBV alone causes the cancer.

EBV has also been found in some B-cell lymphomas occurring in AIDS patients, and in nasopharyngeal cancers in Cantonese Chinese. In this latter group, viral titers can be used for screening high risk populations.

Cervical cancer has many hallmarks of a sexually transmitted disease. Both herpes simplex virus II and human papilloma virus types 16 and 18 have been implicated. There is no direct causal relationship. Good hygiene and the use of measures (e.g. condoms) to prevent sexually transmitted disease may help prevent cervical cancer.

Hepatitis virus is strongly associated with hepatoma. It appears that initiated cells are caused to divide under the stimulus of the virus, and malignant clones are selected. One of the most promising preventive measures for cancer worldwide is the use of hepatitis B vaccine which protects about 90% of previously uninfected people. Hepatoma is one of the most common cancers in the world.

The cancers that occur in AIDS (e.g. Kaposi's sarcoma, non-Hodgkin's and Hodgkin's lymphomas, and oral squamous cell cancers) may well be related to viruses. Preventive measures like "safe sex" (e.g. through the use of condoms, spermicidals, and abstinence), the elimination of needle sharing among addicts, and testing of blood donors will help diminish the ravages of this disease. The great hope, however, is for a vaccine against the causative agent, HIV.

Chapter 5

Screening for Cancer: Concepts and Specific Strategies

Two important movements in medicine today are disease prevention (health maintenance) and cost containment emphasizing efficiency of work-up and care. Sometimes these movements seem at odds, especially when reviewing screening tests for chronic diseases. Can screening recommendations decrease deaths from cancer? Are they cost effective? How does one optimize their performance?

There are few randomized controlled trials showing that mortality is reduced or survival increased by screening. One very important trial, though, is the Health Insurance Plan of New York (the "HIP" study), which clearly showed that mammography and breast physical exam lengthened survival by 30–40% in those screened. Originally, the benefit was confined to women older than 50, but recent data even shows survival benefits of 24% in those women between 40 and 50. Even without many trials definitely proving benefit, sophisticated mathematical models have been produced, using the available data, and they show the potential benefits. Dr. David Eddy generated the data listed in Table 5.1, showing the likelihood that screening will reduce mortality, and the degree of this reduction for certain screening tests in certain cancers. For some cancers (i.e., those of the lung, ovary, and endometrium), there is a good chance of a survival benefit; but the magnitude of this is very small, while for other cancers, the magnitude of reduction is significant (i.e., colon, breast, and cervix).

The characteristics of a cancer that would prove favorable for screening are listed in Table 5.2. There should be a poor prognosis when the cancer

Table 5.1
Benefits of Screening

	Probability of a Screening Test Reducing Mortality	Magnitude of the Benefit
Ovarian cancer	35%	3%
Endometrial cancer	69%	11%
Lung cancer	60%	2%
Breast cancer		
Physical exam and mammography <50	80%	29%
Self exam	80%	15%
Physical exam and mammography >50	94%	38%
Colon cancer		
Stool blood test	82%	18%
Sigmoidoscope	87%	36%
Cervical cancer		
Pap smear	87%	88%

Table 5.2
Characteristics of a Cancer Favorable for Screening

1. Poor prognosis in symptomatic stage.
2. High prevalence in population screened.
3. Detectable presymptomatic stage.
4. Improved prognosis of cancers found by screening.
5. Consensus on efficacy of treatment of early disease.
6. Test must be available.

is treated after symptoms develop. This applies to most cancers, but there are notable exceptions (e.g., the low grade lymphomas). There should also be a high prevalence in the population screened; consideration of risk factors is thus important in selecting the population for testing.

The screening test itself must meet certain criteria. Sensitivity, specificity, and predictive value are defined in Table 5.3. To illustrate, Tables

5.4 and 5.5 list two examples with sensitivity of 80% (that is, four of five cancers will have a positive test) and specificity of 99% (that is, 99 of 100 without the disease will have a negative test). These numbers are well within the range of what is actually seen with many screening tests, such as mammography. Note how the predictive value can be influenced by the population assessed.

Table 5.3
Sensitivity, Specificity and Predictive Value

| | Disease Status | |
	Present	Absent
Positive test	A	C
Test Negative test	B	D

$$\text{Sensitivity} = \frac{A}{A + B}$$

$$\text{Specificity} = \frac{D}{C + D}$$

$$\text{Predictive value of a positive test} = \frac{A}{A + C}$$

Table 5.4
Screening Test Example A

Sensitivity = 80%
Specificity = 99%
Prevalence of the disease = 300/100,000

	Present	Absent
Positive test	240	997
Negative test	60	98,703

$$\text{Predictive value of a positive test} = \frac{240}{240 + 997} = 19\%$$

Table 5.5
Screening Test Example B

Sensitivity = 80%
Specificity = 99%
Prevalence of the disease = 50/100

	Present	Absent
Positive test	400	5
Negative test	100	495

Predictive value of a positive test = 98.8%

To improve the sensitivity, follow the directions for the test as closely as possible. To improve the predictive value, apply the test to a population with a higher prevalence of the disease you are looking for (i.e., people with risk factors).

Critics of screening often involve the lead-time and length-time biases to discount the effects of screening. The lead-time bias means that by screening you may detect cancers earlier, before they would usually present, but even so, the patients survive the same length of time. You have deceived yourself that by identifying this "lead-time," things look better, but in reality, the survival is to the same point. This has been definitely disproven for breast cancer. Women whose cancers were detected by screening *do* live longer.

The length-time bias means that results look better because the more slowly growing, more favorable tumors are those most likely to be diagnosed by screening, while the more rapidly fatal cancers either escape the screen, present in intervals between screenings, or are so biologically aggressive that screening doesn't help. Again, this is not the case for breast cancer where the best studies have been done.

The optimal timing between screenings and the time at which to begin them are other aspects of the tests for which there is not much data. Relying on mathematical models, and extrapolations from the best data available, various national societies have devised recommendations thought to be the most cost-effective.

The following screening measures are recommended by the National Cancer Institute and the American Cancer Society:

A cancer-related checkup:

• every 3 years for those 20–40 years of age.

• every year for those 40 and over.

The checkup should always include health counseling (such as tips on quitting smoking) and examinations for cancer of the thyroid, testes, prostate, mouth, ovaries, skin and lymph nodes.

In particular:

• Ages 20–40—For breast cancer, an examination by a physician every three years, a self-exam every month, and one baseline breast mammogram between the ages of 35 and 39. For cervical cancer, women who are or have been sexually active, or have reached age 18, should have an annual Pap test and pelvic examination. After a woman has had three or more consecutive satisfactory normal annual examinations, the Pap test may be performed less frequently at the discretion of her physician.

• Ages 40 and over—For breast cancer, an exam every year by a health professional, a self-exam every month, and a mammogram every 1–2 years for those 40–49, every year for those 50 and over. For cervical cancer, women who are or have been sexually active, or have reached age 18 years, should have an annual Pap test and pelvic examination. After a woman has had three or more consecutive satisfactory normal annual examinations, the Pap test may be performed less frequently at the discretion of her physician. For women at risk, an endometrial tissue sample at menopause should be taken. For colon and rectum cancer, a digital rectal exam every year after 40, and a stool blood test every year after 40 as well as a proctoscopic exam every 3–5 years after two initial negative tests one year apart.

Some people are at higher risk for certain cancers and may need testing more frequently.

These recommendations are not universally accepted, though they certainly are a reasonable basis with which to start thinking about secondary cancer prevention. The frequency of the proposed screening will certainly involve some expense, and it will/may also generate "false positive" screening results, leading to "unnecessary" work-ups, with their consequent expense and morbidity.

BREAST CANCER

Breast cancer is the most common cancer in women, but lung cancer has recently overtaken it as a cause of cancer death. Screening for breast cancer really works—many studies have shown a decrease in mortality of 30–40%. Until recently, this was felt to be confined to women over 50, but recent data shows benefit also in the 40–49 age group.

The recommendations of the ACS are listed above. On June 27, 1989, 10 other medical organizations announced their agreement on the recommendations for breast cancer screening (the American College of Radiology, The American Academy of Family Physicians, the American Association of Women Radiologists, the AMA, the American Osteopathic College of Radiology, the American Society of Internal Medicine, the American Society for Therapeutic Radiology, the College of American Pathologists, the NCI, and the National Medical Association).

There are three important concepts in screening for breast cancer (and of course, in many other cancers):

1. The predictive value of a positive test can be greatly increased by applying the test to a population with a high prevalence of the disease (i.e., those with risk factors; see Risk Factors in Chapter 2).

2. The sensitivity and specificity of a test can be greatly influenced by how well it is performed. The literature reports sensitivities between 50 and 90% for mammography. Attention to technique and detail, and use of stateof-the-art equipment can maximize test performances.

3. What we do in practice is not truly screening, but case finding. We apply the test to people who come under our care, and this may be a different population than the screening concept of "all" women getting the test.

Mathematical models have shown the importance of the breast exam. Models show that *two-thirds* of the benefit of a screening program *can* come from the properly done physical exam, especially in a case-finding situation. The problem is that we as physicians often do a cursory, incomplete exam and/or we are unsure of our fingers' ability to detect cancer. House officers should go to a "breast screening" clinic if their institution has one, or arrange for one of the skilled surgeons or mammographers to demonstrate for them the proper breast exam.

The second major recommendation for detection of breast cancer is breast self-exam (BSE). Women who practice BSE detect cancers at earlier stages. The problem is that not many women, even after a cancer has been removed from the other breast, practice this technique. Disincentives include the patient's distrust of her own judgment, the discomfort of the exam, and especially the fear of finding cancer with all its possible sequellae. If we can use educators' methods to teach and encourage the use of BSE, perhaps more of our patients would practice it. The ACS has many trained volunteers who help motivate women to do the BSE. As above, it may be worthwhile to arrange for one of the surgeons, the staff of the "breast clinic" or an ACS "expert" to come to a conference to teach housestaff how to teach BSE.

The third and most controversial recommendation is the mammogram. There is no question that mammography detects the earliest cancers, but why is it not practiced more? Only 42% of women over 50 have ever had a mammogram, while only 11% of physicians surveyed by the ACS in 1984 follow the recommended guidelines. There are three major reasons: fear of radiation, availability of equipment, and most importantly, cost. Fear of radiation has been overdone in the popular press. The risk of developing cancer is minimal, and the benefits outweigh the risks. The risk of dying from breast cancer from a mammogram would be equal to the risk of dying from driving a car 100 miles, riding in an airplane cross country, or riding a bike ten miles.

Mammographic equipment is improving all the time, providing better images with less radiation. To improve the sensitivity of a test, the equipment should be as good as possible, the technicians must be careful in their adherence to appropriate procedures, and the film reader should be skillful and experienced in the pitfalls of interpretation. Mammography is not a perfect test. The usual sensitivity is about around 80%, and given the prevalence of the disease, the predictive value of a positive test is about 10–20%. This means that only one out of every five to ten biopsies will actually show cancer, and in many screening studies this is the actual case.

There are currently at least 7000 mammography units in the U.S. The American College of Radiology is running a voluntary accreditation program, and as of July, 1989, 1257 units had been reviewed. Of those reviewed, about two-thirds passed the standard tests, and the ACR is working with the other centers to improve the quality. An ACR accredited center will be known to be of good quality.

This leaves cost as the major stumbling block. Mammography is expensive, especially when done in a diagnostic department as a case finding situation, instead of at a lower cost in a government supported screening program. Furthermore, most insurance policies do not cover screening mammograms. (However, this seems to be changing.)

These are the negative aspects, but mammography is a good and important test. If there are risk factors, especially family history, a prior cancer, or a history of atypical hyperplasia on a previous biopsy, the American Cancer Society (ACS) recommendations should be followed. What should you do if there are no risk factors (this is where 75% of breast cancers come from)? In the best of all worlds, the recommendations of the ACS would produce the greatest benefit. But, given the availability of equipment and cost considerations, a practical approach would be to: 1) perform as good a physical exam as possible each year; 2) teach BSE; 3) if you are not sure of your exam (or if there is anything suspicious), order a mammogram. If possible, try to do mammograms every one to two years in women over 40 with or without minor risk factors, and emphasize to them the importance of physical exam and breast self-exam.

Three other points need to be made about mammography:

1. Mammography and physical exam are complementary. If you feel a suspicious area, but the mammogram is negative, it should be biopsied.

2. If the mammographer tells you he is sure there is a cancer, but the biopsy is negative, make sure the right area was biopsied.

3. Remember, if there is a lump, then what is being done is a diagnostic mammogram. All women with suspicious lumps should have a mammogram, and it is recommended that women who will undergo augmentive or reductive breast surgery should also have a preoperative study.

The subject of mammography is reviewed in detail in a recent article by Eddy (*Annals of Internal Medicine* 111:389–399, 1989). He has developed useful tables that could be helpful to the practitioner discussing the risks and benefits of the procedure. More than 80% of women surveyed by the NCI have said they would get a mammogram if their physicians had advised them to do this.

It is incumbent on us to work to decrease the death rate from cancer of the breast. The NCI wants us to get 80% of women in compliance with the screening recommendations by the year 2000.

COLORECTAL CANCER

Risk factors for colon cancer are listed in Chapter 2. Special screening programs may have to be suggested for high risk patients. Consult with the gastroenterology service at your hospital for local recommendations.

For the general population, three screening tests are recommended: the rectal exam, the stool blood test, and proctosigmoidoscopy. Only about 10% of cancers can be detected by the rectal exam, because cancers are now occurring more proximally in the colon. There have been no studies to date proving that screening by rectal exam increases survival, but the exam is safe and easily performed and should be part of the recommended general physical exam in all patients over age 40.

The second test is the stool blood test, which should also be performed yearly after age 40. The Hemoccult-2® is the test most commonly used. This test detects 2–4 ml of blood per 100 gm of stool, an amount about 50% greater than is normally lost each day.

The patient must prepare for the test by avoiding red meat, aspirin, nonsteroidal anti-inflammatory drugs, and vitamin C and by increasing the intake of roughage. The test should not be taken if there has been recent epistaxis. Two specimens should be obtained from each of three consecutive stools and brought to the physician immediately, since a delay of four days may turn a weakly positive test negative. Any blue color seen on the slide within 30 seconds after applying the developer is considered positive. There is a quality control area on most slides. A drop of developing solution placed there should turn blue. This not only gives the physician an indicator of the blue color he is looking for, but also tests the slide quality itself.

There are currently ongoing controlled trials on the use of the stool blood test, which are not yet far enough along to show differences between groups. These studies should be mature in the next few years and should help settle the issue of whether occult blood screening for colon cancer really does work. The U.S. Preventive Services Task Force has recently published their report, and they say: "There is insufficient evidence to recommend for or against fecal occult blood testing or sigmoidoscopy as effective screening tests for colorectal cancer in asymptomatic persons. There are also inadequate grounds for discontinuing this form of screening where it is currently practiced or for withholding it from persons who request it. It may be clinically prudent to offer screening to persons aged 50 and older with known risk factors for colorectal cancer. (from Guide to Clinical Preventive Services, Report of the U.S. Preventive Services Task Force)

Despite lack of "proof" that screening works, data from many uncontrolled trials show that the stool blood test is well accepted by both patients and physicians. There is a 2–5% rate of positive tests, with from 30–50% of positives having either polyps or cancer. The predictive value of a positive test for cancer is actually 8%. Cancers detected by hemoccults are more likely to be early stage lesions.

Problems with the stool blood test include the rate of false negatives. Careful studies have shown that 72% of polyps and 24% of cancers are without blood for the three-day test period. Another problem is in the rate of false positives. Since 30–50% of lesions are due to neoplasia, 50–70% are not. Work-up usually defines some type of pathology, but it may be costly and uncomfortable for the patient.

There are many new and more sensitive tests becoming available, but currently they are too costly and time-consuming for recommended use. Slides like the Hemoccult-2® are currently the best choice, but in the future, other test kits may succeed this relatively inexpensive and nonspecific test.

The third recommendation is proctosigmoidoscopy. Two yearly exams are recommended after age 50 and if negative, repeated every 3–5 years thereafter. The incidence of rectal cancers is greatly reduced in screened populations. Proctoscopy discovers a cancer in only one of every 500 exams of average risk patients. However, removal of polyps, the premalignant lesions, greatly reduces risk.

Problems with proctoscopy include patient discomfort, physician reluctance to do an uncomfortable exam, the risk of bowel perforation, and especially cost. The rigid proctoscope which is in most common use, is often not inserted to its full length. The depth of insertion is usually between 13 to 16 cm.

Flexible fiberoptic scopes have recently been utilized and are both more easily tolerated by the patient and able to facilitate detection of more lesions. A 60 cm sigmoidoscope is currently in use, but this should be used only by trained physicians. Recently, a 35 cm flexible sigmoidoscope has been introduced. This is easier to use, especially by physicians without the special training.

One of the major hurdles to the use of sigmoidoscopy is cost. It is the most costly colorectal screening procedure, and flexible sigmoidoscopes are even more costly. As in breast cancer, people at risk should be screened. For others, one has to weigh the potential benefits of discovering and removing polyps and cancer against cost and inconvenience. The author feels that the recommendation of sigmoidoscopic examinations every five years after 50 years of age is reasonable. Remember, there is no effective therapy after dissemination has occurred.

Just as the breast exam and mammography are complementary procedures for breast cancer diagnosis, so too are hemoccult testing and proctoscopy complementary for colon cancer screening. Of course, patients with symptoms or positive stool blood tests should be thoroughly examined.

CERVICAL CANCER

The control of cervical cancer is a success story for screening. Cervical cancer is the second most common malignancy of the female reproductive tract, affecting 2% of women. There are 16,000 cases per year of invasive cervical cancer in the United States, and 45,000 causes of in situ cancer. Over the past 20 years, through the use of the Papanicolaou (Pap) test, preinvasive cancer is being more commonly diagnosed. Because of this, there is less invasive cancer found, and hence a dramatic lowering of the death rate.

The risk factors for cervical cancer are reviewed in Chapter 2. It is known that cervical cancer represents a continuous spectrum of epithelial changes that occur over time. The earliest phase is called cervical intraepithelial neoplasia (CIN) grade I (or mild dysplasia). This can be diagnosed when undifferentiated atypical cells occupy one-third of the epithelium. In CIN grade II (moderate dysplasia) the cells occupy threequarters of the epithelium. With CIN grade III (severe dysplasia or carcinoma in situ), the cells occupy the whole epithelium. The next phase is frank invasion, which may be micro or macroscopic. Prognosis becomes worse with more severe changes in the spectrum. A 100% cure rate can be attained in CIN grades I–III.

Improving the sensitivity of a test can improve its usefulness. In the literature, the sensitivity of the Pap test has been reported to be as low as 67%; simple attention to detail can improve this up to 90%. Factors leading to decreased sensitivity include poor preparation of the patient, examination technique, laboratory technique, and follow-up on positive reports. The patient should be encouraged not to douche or have a tub bath for 24 hours prior to the exam. Lubricant should not be used for the exam. Since cancer begins in the transformation zone between the glandular and squamous epithelium, samples must be taken from there. Often, this area is not visible, especially in elderly patients. Some examiners recommend the use of a moistened saline swab passed through the cervical os, especially if the zone is not clearly seen. The specimen should be spread thinly and evenly on the slide and fixed immediately with the spray can of fixative held about one foot away. The slide should be carefully labeled. The laboratory should be an integrated reporting system, with physicians being familiar with the terms used on reported results.

Another way to optimize cervical cancer screening is to optimize the timing. Because of the usual long natural history of the disease, both mathematical models and much experience support taking Pap smears every three years, after two negative studies done one year apart. (However, most gynecologists still favor more frequent exams.) Routine Pap smears should begin when sexual activity commences and continue through age 60. A practical approach would be to do yearly smears for high risk women, and Pap smears every three years for all others.

The ACS does recommend a yearly pelvic exam. Careful palpation of the uterus and ovaries is essential. Remember, if the ovary is palpable postmenopausally, this suggests possible ovarian cancer. Risks for endometrial cancer include age greater than 40, obesity, a history of anovulatory cycles, infertility, and the use of estrogen hormones. In this group, consideration should be given to doing endometrial tissue sampling after menopause. Abnormal uterine bleeding warrants thorough evaluation. Also, the gynecologic exam is an excellent time to emphasize health-related issues, such as breast self-examination, and modifying risk factors in general.

PROSTATE CANCER

Prostate cancer is the third leading cause of cancer deaths in men.

The key to early diagnosis is the rectal exam, which is recommended yearly after age 40. It is suggested that nodules as small as 2 mm can be felt by the experienced finger. I prefer to examine patients in the standing position with elbows resting on the examination table, toes pointed inward, and knees bent. The examining finger should be well-lubricated and gently passed through the sphincter to reduce spasm. Examine the gland systematically from left to right. Some suggest bending the tip of the finger slightly, which allows for more discrimination of nodules deeper in the substance of the gland, or having the patient Valsalva during the exam, which brings the gland toward the examining finger.

Some have suggested that the recent advances in assaying acid phosphate by RIA will make it a valuable screening test in asymptomatic men. However, applying the actual numbers obtained for sensitivity and specificity of this test to the population in the United States known to have the highest prevalence, it was found that only 0.44%, or one patient in 244, with a positive test would have prostate cancer. Rectal exam remains the key test.

Several other tests are now being evaluated. These include the assay for prostate-specific antigen and trans-rectal ultrasound. The former is like the acid phosphatase test and at the present time is not specific enough for screening. Transrectal ultrasound is an important technologic advance, but its exact role is not yet defined. It seems best used with a battery of other tests, including the rectal to define the extent of prostate cancer in the gland.

MELANOMA

Malignant melanoma accounts for only 1% of cancer deaths, though the incidence of this disease is rising faster than any other neoplasm other than lung cancer in women. Risk factors for melanoma are listed in Chapter 2. Recently, a high risk familial syndrome, dysplastic nevus syndrome, has been recognized. Families are being increasingly identified by attention to pigmented lesions. It is important to recognize dysplastic nevi because the lifetime risk in family members approaches 100% and early detection can produce cure. An informative color atlas has been published, and every practitioner should study the details given (*N Engl J Med* 312:91–97, 1985).

During a physical exam, every mole a patient has should be inspected. A normal Caucasian has about 15–20 moles. The ACS suggests that early warning signs for melanoma should include changes in size, bleeding, or ulceration in a mole. These are often later signs of melanomas, and occur where invasion and metastasis are more likely. The earliest signs are given in Table 5.6 and include variegated color, especially shades of red, white, and blue, and the presence of a notch or an irregular border. Normal moles are usually smaller than 1 cm, while melanomas are more likely to be larger. Melanomas should be diagnosable before deep invasion has occurred by simple attention to the detail of a patient's pigmented lesions.

OTHER CANCERS

Tragically, the incidence of lung cancer continues to increase worldwide. It has long been the leading cause of cancer death in men in the U.S., and recently has become the leading cause of cancer death among women. Attempts at early diagnosis by frequent chest x-rays in asymptomatic, high risk men have not been successful in increasing survival. Recently, physicians at the Mayo Clinic, Johns Hopkins, and Memorial-Sloan Kettering have screened high risk patients by frequent sputum cytologies plus x-rays, and although the survival may be slightly increased, the benefit is marginal and expensive. Many feel the money would be much more usefully spent in trying to influence smoking habits. Lung cancer is largely a preventable disease, and physicians should attempt to influence individual patients to stop or never to start smoking. Probably even more importantly, physicians should help to develop educational programs in

Table 5.6
Signs of Melanoma[a]

Early Signs
1. Variegated color—especially shades of red, white or blue.
2. Irregular border and an angular indentation or notch.
Later Signs
3. Increase in size or change in color
4. Irregular elevation of the surface
Late Signs
5. Bleeding, ulceration, pain

---

[a] From Del Med J 59(2): 1987.

their communities on the dangers of smoking, and influence legislators, insurers, and employers to foster anti-smoking activity.

Head and neck cancer is another smoking related cancer. Other risk factors include alcohol use, poor oral hygiene, and smokeless tobacco use. Recently, the latter has become increasingly popular, especially among young athletes. Many dentists are currently doing a wonderful job of screening for oral cancer. Physicians often do a cursory, superficial exam of the oral cavity. Attention to detail may help in recognition of early oral cancers and premalignant lesions. Special attention should be given to heavy smokers, alcohol abusers, and patients who use smokeless tobacco products.

Self-examination for young males has been suggested as a means of early detection for testicular cancer. There often is a long delay between a patient noticing a testicular mass and his seeking medical attention. Heightened awareness of the curability of testicular cancer may be able to lessen the fear of a patient with a testicular mass.

In other parts of the world, screening is done for gastric cancer (Japan), esophageal cancer (China), nasopharyngeal cancer (by E.B. virus titers in Cantonese Chinese), and hepatoma (by alpha-fetoprotein levels, in Africa and China).

The most perfect cancer for which to screen is medullary carcinoma of the thyroid in the familial form. The prevalence is 50% in family members, since its inheritance is autosomal dominant, and there is not only a good marker for the disease (i.e., calcitonin levels) but also a good provocative test (calcium or pentagastrin infusions) to stimulate production of calcitonin in family members with cancer but normal baseline calcitonin.

SUMMARY

1. Many cancers may be preventable.

2. Primary prevention is the best, most cost effective way to prevent cancer.

3. The most important thing we can do to prevent cancer is to get our patients not to smoke.

4. Secondary prevention (screening) is also effective.

5. Follow recommendations of the ACS listed on page 5 and 6 of this chapter (as written).

Chapter 6

Approach to the Patient: Evaluation, Diagnosis, Staging, and Questions about Treatment

INTRODUCTION

Care of the patient with cancer involves an integrated evaluation of the patient's general health (patient factors), characteristics and nature of the cancer (tumor factors), and therapeutic options (treatment factors).

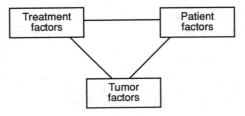

The patient with cancer has an autonomous illness whose salient features include the ability to metastasize and the ability to destroy normal tissue. These features may result in compromised vital organ function. Development of symptoms such as pain in one or more areas, cough, and problems such as bowel or duct obstruction provide some of the clues or keys toward patient evaluation.

At the time of diagnosis the patient may be asymptomatic. A painless neck lump, or abnormal preemployment chest x-ray may be the first hint of cancer. The majority of patients, however, are symptomatic. The patient may be symptomatic from tissue destruction at the primary site, an area of metastasis, or both. In addition, he may have developed a paraneoplastic syndrome, or remote effect of cancer, not directly due to the tumor mass itself.

The house officer may be involved with patients with cancer at the time of initial diagnosis and therapy, at the time of cancer relapse, during the time of treatment complication, or in some patients, during the final weeks or days of life. Evaluation of the patient with cancer at any of these times involves consideration of patient, tumor, and treatment factors, past and present.

This chapter will address the basics of each of these factors, the therapeutic index as it applies to patients with cancer, and some questions about therapy.

PATIENT FACTORS

Patient factors can be thought of as one's general state of health, noncancer related conditions, and alterations of health due to cancer.

1. General
   a. Age and gender
   b. Nutritional status, weight, and change in weight
   c. Performance status (PS). A statement or measurement of a patient's ambulatory capacity, symptoms, and need for assistance. PS is usually described by one of two scales: Karnofsky, and Zubrod (or ECOG: Eastern Cooperative Oncology Group). Karnofsky rates PS on a scale of 100% (best) to 0% (dead). The ECOG scale of 0 (best) to 4 (poorest) is easier to remember.

ECOG PS	Description
0	Normal activity
1	Symptoms but ambulatory and able to carry out daily activities
2	Out of bed more than 50% of time, occasionally needs assistance.
3	In bed more than 50% of time, needs skilled care.
4	100% Bedridden

Performance status is an important determinant of prognosis and response to therapy.

2. Comorbid conditions and treatment history
   a. Cardiovascular
   b. Pulmonary
   c. Renal
   d. Gastrointestinal
   e. Endocrine
   f. Dermatologic
   g. Musculoskeletal
   h. Nervous system
   i. Hematopoietic

3. Emotional factors. This includes the patient's past emotional or psychiatric history, if any, as well as his emotional state at the time of evaluation.

4. Symptoms and signs. Questions that should be asked include: 1) At the time of diagnosis: what symptoms and signs are due to cancer? 2) During therapy: what symptoms and signs are due to cancer and what symptoms and signs are due to treatment toxicity? 3) After therapy, what symptoms and signs are due to cancer progression (if this occurs), and which are due to late toxicities of therapy?

TUMOR FACTORS

Tumor factors include the tissue diagnosis, extent of disease (stage), tempo of disease, determination of resectability, and consideration of known responsiveness to radiation therapy and systemic therapy.

1. Diagnosis. Once an abnormality has been identified, a *tissue diagnosis* is sought. A tissue diagnosis is the cornerstone on which all further evaluation and treatment decisions are based. A tissue diagnosis can be thought of as consisting of tissue procurement and tissue identification.
   a. Tissue procurement. Generally, we would like to sample tissue that is the most accessible and likely to yield results with the least complicated procedure. There are two types of diagnostic material:

1) Single cells or clusters of malignant cells found in body fluids or exfoliated from organs. Cytology specimens in body fluids include those from pleural and pericardial effusions, ascites, and cerebrospinal fluid. Cytology specimens exfoliated from organs include those obtained in sputum, urine, and cervical Pap smears.

2) Tissue samples obtained by endoscopic or surgical biopsy. An *incisional* biopsy involves removing a small piece of a lesion. An excisional biopsy removes the entire lesion.

b. Tissue identification. Exfoliated cells or bioposy specimens are sent to the pathology laboratory for standard preparation and stains such as H and E, cytology stains, and immunohistochemical studies. When indicated, material may be sent for estrogen and progesterone receptors, flow cytometry, and electron microscopy. These studies yield the histopathology of the malignancy, that is, the tumor type, classification, and grade.

1) Type:
   a) Carcinoma
   b) Sarcoma
   c) Germ cell tumor
   d) Lymphoma
   e) Glioma

2) Classification: or subtype of the above five malignancies. For example, is the carcinoma a squamous, adeno, large cell, small cell, or undifferentiat ed carcinoma?

3) Grade: Grade describes the degree to which a malignant tumor resembles normal tissue. A tumor containing many cellular and architectural features of normal tissue is called well differentiated, or low grade. A tumor containing few features of normal tissue is called poorly differentiated, high grade, or anaplastic.

   The grade of a tumor plays a role in prognosis and in treatment decisions in the following tumor types:
   a) Gliomas
   b) Soft tissue sarcoma
   c) Ovarian cancer
   d) Prostate cancer
   e) Malignant lymphoma
   f) Bladder cancer
   g) Endometrial cancer

2. Stage. Once an abnormality is identified and a tissue diagnosis made, staging or determination of extent of disease is undertaken.

   a. Reasons for staging: 1) to define the extent of disease in order to make treatment decisions, define the objective of therapy, and determine prognosis; 2) measure and follow the results of therapy; and 3) standardize the description of extent of disease in order to accurately compare results of investigational or standard therapy, of different tumor types among different institutions.

   b. Staging systems:

     1) TNM (system of the American Joint Committee on Cancer: AJCC). This system is used for most types of cancers.

     T = *primary tumor* characteristics such as location, size, and adjacent tissue involvement (T_1 through T_4).

     N = local-regional *lymph node* involvement with tumor (N_0 = no involvement; $N_1 N_2 N_3$ = various increasing degrees of involvement).

     M = Presence or absence of metastasis and their location.

     In the TNM system, different cancers have different definitions of T,N, and M. Once a T,N and M is defined for an individual's cancer, a stage is assigned.

     2) Other staging systems:

       a. Ann Arbor: for malignant lymphomas and Hodgkin's disease.

       b. UICC: International Union Against Cancer, for breast cancer.

       c. FIGO: International Federation of Gynecology and Obstetrics, for ovarian cancer.

   c. Staging methods. Staging always starts with a careful and complete *history and physical examination.* In addition, tests ordered to determine extent of disease depend on: 1) tumor type; 2) symptoms and location of signs; and 3) whether or not the patient is being considered for an investigational treatment protocol which may have strict staging requirements.

3. Tempo of disease. As important as knowing tumor type and stage of disease is the clinical determination of disease tempo. Tempo of disease describes the rate of growth, or the rate of spread, or how quickly a tumor has incapacitated an individual.

   a. The main value in assessing disease tempo is in decision making about how quickly treatment needs to be started. Gauging disease tempo will define the "window of opportunity" or the window of time within which to work prior to starting emergency therapy and anti-cancer therapy.

b. Tempo of disease may be judged by: 1) *severity* of symptoms and signs; 2) *duration* of symptoms and signs; and 3) in the case of disease recurrence or progression, the interval of time between first diagnosis and treatment, and the time of first recurrence (sometimes referred to as the *disease free interval* or relapse free interval).

c. Aggressive or quick tempo disease may cause severe symptoms or signs over a short period of time (days to weeks, or sometimes hours), or be characterized by a short (less than 1 or 2 years) disease-free interval. Indolent or slowly growing tumors may cause only mild symptoms or signs over a long period of time (weeks to months), or recur after a long (greater than 2–5 years) disease-free interval.

d. Keep in mind that not all quick tempo or aggressive malignancies carry a poor prognosis.

4. Determination of resectability. The clinical determination of whether a malignant tumor can be completely removed with a surgical procedure (resectable tumor) is made by the surgical oncologist and internist. The resectable or unresectable status of a patient with a malignant tumor is primarily judged by knowing the tumor type, stage of disease, and physiologic status of the patient.

5. The final tumor factor is the inherent sensitivity or insensitivity of the tumor to radiation therapy (RT) and systemic anticancer therapies (hormonal therapy and antineoplastic chemotherapy). Knowledge of responsivity to RT or systemic therapy is gained through Phase II and Phase III clinical trials. The results of these trials are published in peer-reviewed journals or are summarized and explained in textbooks.

TREATMENT FACTORS

Treatment factors, or the major types of available anti-cancer therapy, fall into two large catagories: local treatment modalities and systemic treatment modalities. Local treatments include surgery and radiation therapy.

1. Systemic treatment. Systemic treatment modalities include antineo
   plastic chemotherapy, hormonal therapy, and immunologic therapy.
   a. When using systemic therapy, it is important to keep in mind the
      following points as they relate to the drug or drugs being used:
      1) Drug classification and mechanism of action
      2) Pharmacokinetics and pharmacodynamics
      3) Antitumor activity
      4) Toxicity
      5) Drug interaction
      6) Principles of drug use
   b. Antineoplastic chemotherapy. The chemotherapy drugs are natu-
      rally occurring or synthetic compounds that kill cells (cytoxic) or
      inhibit the proliferation of cells by a variety of mechanisms. The
      action of these drugs, however, is nonspecific in that many normal
      cell populations are affected.
   c. Hormonal therapy. Hormonal therapy or hormonal "manipulation"
      can be either additive or ablative.
      1) Additive:
         a) Corticosteroids
         b) Estrogens
         c) Progestins
         d) Androgens
      2) Ablative:
         a) Antiestrogens
         b) Antiandrogens
         c) Gonadotropin analogues
         d) Oophorectomy and orchiectomy are local treatments having
            a systemic hormonal effect
   d. Chemotherapy and hormonal therapy drugs are either commercially
      available or investigational, that is, only available for use on certain
      protocols or at certain institutions.
   e. Immunologic therapy. Immunologic therapy currently involves the
      use of lymphokines, lymphokine activated-killer cells, and mono-
      clonal antibodies, to mention just a few.

THE THERAPEUTIC INDEX

The therapeutic index (TI) is a comparison or ratio of the effect of therapy on the patient (toxicity) to the effect of therapy on the patient's malignancy (efficacy).

$$TI = \frac{Toxicity}{Efficacy} = \frac{Effect\ of\ Patient}{Effect\ on\ Tumor}$$

Nowhere in the arena of disease and therapeutics does consideration of the therapeutic index become as important as it does with the use of cytotoxic chemotherapy or ionizing radiation for the treatment of cancer. For antineoplastic chemotherapy and radiation therapy, the TI can be expressed in terms of dose.

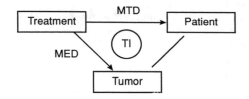

$$TI = \frac{MTD}{MED} = \frac{Maximum\ Tolerated\ Dose}{Minimum\ Effective\ Dose} = \frac{Toxicity}{Efficacy}$$

For most medications the MED is much smaller than the MTD; that is, the desired effect can be achieved with no, or minimum, toxicity. An example would be use of aspirin or acetaminophen for mild pain. In this example, the TI is high.

For antineoplastic chemotherapy, however, the MED is frequently the same as the MTD; that is, the dose causing tumor shrinkage is also causing severe side effects. In this case, the TI is low or close to one.

QUESTIONS ABOUT THERAPY

Once the patient has been evaluated, a tissue diagnosis known and, either during staging or after staging is completed, questions and decisions about therapy are entertained. The following questions should be addressed during inpatient rounds and in the ambulatory setting about each patient.

1. **Am I going to treat the patient or not?** The first decision is to recommend anti-cancer therapy or no anti-cancer therapy. Perhaps the most difficult decision of all is to recommend no therapy. This can occur in a number of settings. The first example is the elderly patient with a dementia syndrome unrelated to his cancer who does not understand his disease, treatment options, and side effects. It may in this setting be appropriate to recommend no anti-cancer therapy. A second setting is in a patient who has already undergone multiple anti-cancer therapies and continues to have disease progression, or is dying. The decision to recommend no further anticancer therapy, that is, to stop anti-cancer therapy, is appropriate in many of these instances. Another setting involves the patient with a newly diagnosed cancer that has a long natural history and is not causing any problems (e.g., follicular lymphoma, or chronic lymphocytic leukemia). In this setting, it is usually appropriate to recommend no anti-cancer therapy at the outset, but to wait until indicated in the future.

2. **What is the object of therapy?** If the decision to treat the patient with anti-cancer therapy has been made, the first question is: what is the object of therapy? The object of therapy will be either to cure the patient of his malignancy or to *palliate*. To cure an individual of his malignancy means to eliminate all evidence of disease for the duration of his life. To palliate means to relieve symptoms of the disease without curing the patient. The object of therapy is generally determined by knowledge of the type of malignancy present, stage of disease, age of the patient, the performance status, and the efficacy of treatment modalities.

3. **How am I going to treat the patient?** Surgery, radiation therapy, or systemic therapies, individually or together (combined modality therapy) can be used in the curative or palliative setting. These modalities can be used at the time of diagnosis or at the time of disease progression. The choice of anti-cancer modality depends on the type of malignancy, stage of disease, performance status, and object of therapy.

4. **When am I going to treat the patient?** As important as deciding about treating the patient or not, the object of therapy, and the method of therapy is the question of timing of treatment. That is to say, does the patient need to be treated immediately, or can a few days or weeks go by prior to starting therapy? In addition to the nature of the malignancy

and stage of disease, the tempo of disease is the main factor in determining timing of therapy. Quick tempo or aggressive disease, causing severe symptoms and signs, needs to be addressed and treated quickly.

5. **How long am I going to treat the patient?** The question of duration of anti-cancer therapy is perhaps the most difficult of all. This question applies primarily to those patients whose anti-cancer modality is systemic, i.e. chemotherapy or hormonal therapy. The factors to consider include the type of malignancy, stage of disease, and object of therapy.

CONCLUSION

Patient factors, tumor factors, and treatment factors should be addressed in the patient with cancer both at the time of diagnosis and later, during and after the patient's treatments. Careful integration of these factors will result in optimal patient care.

Chapter 7

Talking to a Patient with Cancer

There is perhaps no more privileged role in medicine than that of a physician who is entrusted with the overall care of a patient with cancer. In training programs, the responsibility (and emotional duress) for oncology care is shared with young physicians and students, who generally are not taught specifically how to communicate with cancer patients. The development of communication skills is typically perfected over time, with memorable triumphs and frustrations.

What makes the physician-patient interaction so unique in oncology relates to the nature of cancer itself and to human perceptions of the cancer process. For many Americans, cancer is a frightening, unpredictable disease that will likely result in suffering, disfigurement, and eventually death. Virtually every adult in our society has experienced the loss of a loved one or an acquaintance to the ravages of cancer. Indeed, those individuals who fare poorly are more visible (or well known) than the fortunate survivors, who often do not wish to publicize their success. It is understandable then how anxious patients may be in their initial encounters with physicians who will care for them; this anxiety will often cloud their ability to comprehend and retain medical information.[1]

The relationship between a physician and a cancer patient has evolved considerably from physician authority and patient passivity to a mutual participation model. In an age when patients insist on more complete understanding of their situation and the potential alternatives, physicians have felt increasing pressure to spend more time with patients, to research new ideas and, most notably, to listen to them. Unfortunately, with the forces of medical economics and productivity ratings impinging on physician behavior, the unique and refreshing human characteristics of a patient may be overlooked—this remains an elemental challenge for caregivers who would be wise to look for patients' strengths and build on them during the course of their disease.

Of the major characteristics an individual with cancer seeks in a physician, a command of medical knowledge is paramount. Not only should the physician be able to discuss in detail the various possibilities appropriate for a given situation, but the options should be presented in an easily intelligible manner. A simple, down-to-earth vocabulary and style are essential elements to patient understanding. Repeated explanations and assessments of patient comprehension are usually necessary to achieve optimal patient management.

Medical prowess, however, includes more facets than straightforward communication; in addition, physicians should be aware of the emotional, cognitive, behavioral, and social problems that cancer patients commonly face.[2] Various strong emotional reactions and fears are universal, and patients should be reassured that they are not abnormal if they ask "stupid questions" or have unusual concerns. Another comfort for cancer patients is the knowledge that their primary physicians are included in decision-making and updates on their course. Experienced physicians and oncology nurses also can anticipate certain misconceptions that frequently torment patients, such as: "chemotherapy that doesn't cause nausea or hair loss isn't working on the tumor," or any "surgery on a tumor is likely to make it spread like wildfire throughout the body."

A caring attitude is a second much sought-after characteristic in a physician. Patients need to know they won't be abandoned, no matter how difficult their plight or bleak their prognosis. Part of the physician's art is imparting a message to the patient that he/she is important as a person and that his/her course has meaning to the physician. Important elements of caring include the capacity to physically touch the patient at appropriate times (a widely appreciated gesture), to show a sense of humor emphasizing that the serious nature of illness is not all-encompassing, and to remember important facets of the patient's life. Patients should be encouraged or given permission to ask questions, share concerns, and express emotions; many feel that they don't know how to ask or that the physician doesn't have the time.[3] A useful exercise for young physicians on rounds is to present a case while speaking in the first person, i.e. to try to put themselves in the patient's plight; this impersonation can give a more human quality to that individual, who may otherwise be considered "a case." If patients perceive a sense of caring by the medical team, they are more likely to adhere to medical recommendations[4] and less likely to experience emotional distress[5]; ultimately, this relationship may decrease demands on the caregivers by avoiding misunderstandings and decreasing stress.

Physicians should preserve honesty and hope in their relationships with cancer patients throughout the various phases of illness. Even if a cure or remission is not likely, patients need to feel that there is some "good time" left where they can find moments of serenity or happiness in their lives. The issue of honesty most often pertains to general information about a particular disease, its course, and prognosis. Obviously, patients will not require the total available fund of knowledge about their particular situation, but each will have his/her needs ranging from much to very little. Thus, a limited but variable amount of information will be appropriate in each case.

Similarly, the need for exactness of a prognosis will vary; some will never inquire and others will want specifics. In this delicate and sensitive area, one needs to feel how directly the patient is approaching the issue, as it is not appropriate (nor considerate) for a physician to announce a prognosis in specific terms unless it is requested first by the patient or serves an extraordinary purpose (e.g. establishing an urgent code status). Generally, if requested, it will be sufficient to give the patient a range of time during which the disease process can reasonably be controlled—the need for a "ballpark" figure is often real, since patients must settle their affairs. A reminder that they may fare much better than average can positively influence the discussion.

The optimal care of an individual with cancer will frequently require a combined effort approach; the talents of an oncologist, an oncology nurse, a primary care physician, a chaplain or other members of the clergy, and visiting nurses at home are all valuable. When adjustments are particularly difficult, a psychiatric referral is often helpful, while support groups, discussions with other individual cancer patients, and hospice organizations alleviate lesser degrees of anxiety and uncertainty.

The final phase of interaction is the period immediately before and including death. The patient and family will usually have more intense needs at this time, including heightened levels of communication. The relationship built over time between patient and physician will facilitate preparations for comfort measures prior to the end of life. Periodic house calls or telephone calls to check on the patient's status can provide immeasurable reassurance at a time when visits to the physician are impractical. In the end, the sense of loss experienced by a physician can often be overcome by the realization that a difference was made, and a person of worth was guided through life's last perils in a satisfactory fashion.

Points to Remember

1. Listen to the patient. Here are some useful points about listening:

   a. Show you want to listen. Be alert; face the person you're talking to. Make eye contact. Lean forward. Be interested.

   b. React with nods, encouragement, and smiles.

   c. Question what you don't understand. Stop talking. Some suggest a "2 second" rule, where you wait at least 2 seconds after the other person is finished to respond. Don't keep interrupting.

   d. Have empathy. Try to put yourself in the other's position.

   e. Get rid of distractions. Try to erase your worries of what the last person you saw said—concentrate on who is with you now.

One special type of listening is called "active listening." You use this when somebody comes to you with a problem—and most of the time this is what your patients will be doing, but it may also happen with your peers, friends, etc. In "active" listening," one tries to feel the emotion or the concern that the other person is telling you and "reflect" it back to him or her. It can be very useful with cancer patients, e.g. a man with known lung cancer comes in very concerned about pain in his arm—the x-ray is normal. One solution might be to say "everything is OK," but with "active listening," the following might be said: "You seem really worried about a recurrence." Active listening is a powerful tool, but it takes time and energy to really "tune in" to another person.

2. Look for what is uniquely human in each patient. Always maintain the ideals and personal values of the patient. Accept people for what they are, and remember, there are no typical terminal patients, only people who happen to be dying. Don't try to turn them into what you would like them to be or to behave like your notion of an ideal patient.

3. Know your stuff, and make the effort to find new information pertinent to your patient. Remember that being good at whatever your task is results in emotional as well as medical benefits for the patient. Make sure that treatments are no worse than the disease they are trying to cure or palliate. Consider carefully the benefits of medical technology versus its tendency to lead to overtreatment or to isolate individuals from their families, homes, and all that gives meaning to their lives or to take away decision making power and dignity.

4. Let the patient know you care. Remember, medicine is a caring profession, not simply the curing of an illness. Of all the attributes of a physician, none is more highly valued by terminal patients than your ability to care. Be consistent in patient contact, and promote a trusting relationship with patients and families. They are counting on your presence. The fear of isolation and the feeling of abandonment can be decreased or increased by you. Be there; make your presence felt at the bedside. Patients don't fear dying as much as dying alone.

5. Hope should not be summarily removed from a patient. There is always something that can be done to improve the quality of a person's life—or death.

6. Rely on the talents of others to assist in the total care of the patient.

7. The little things often mean a great deal to someone facing death. Promote the comfort of the patient. Every aspect of comfort must be sought, not just pain control, but mouth care, hygiene, and nutrition.

8. Find those things (exercise, hobbies, etc.) that you find relaxing and make time for them.

9. Remember #8.

REFERENCES

1. Weisman, A.D., Worden, J.W.: The existential plight in cancer: Significance of the first 100 days. *Int J Psychiatry Med* 7:1, 1976–77.
2. Meyerowitz, B.E., Heinrich, R.L., Coscarelli Schag, C.A.: Helping patients cope with cancer. *Oncology* 3:120, 1989.
3. Messerli, M.L., Garamendi, C., Romano, J.: Breast cancer: Information as a technique of crisis intervention. *Am J Orthopsychiatry* 50:728, 1980.
4. Garrity, T.F.: Medical compliance and clinician-patient relationship: A review. *Soc Sci Med* 15E:215, 1981.
5. Meyerowitz, B.E.: Psychosocial correlates of breast cancer and its treatments. *Psychol Bull* 87:108, 1980.

Chapter 8

Surgical Approach to the Patient

The role of surgery in the management of patients with benign and malignant neoplasms has undergone a great evolution since the first abdominal operation to remove an ovarian tumor was performed in America in 1809 by Ephraim MacDowell. The first era of development of cancer therapy emerged with surgical extirpation as the only modality of treatment for most solid tumors and was greatly facilitated by the introduction of general anesthesia [using ether] by Morton and Long in 1846, and later by a description of the principles of antisepsis presented in the Lancet by Lister in 1867. Encouraged by the advances in anesthesia and improved methods of wound care and infection control, and stimulated by Halsted's principles of 'en bloc resections', the concept of aggressive and extensive surgical removal of most solid tumors expanded. However, as the initial improvement in survival began to plateau, the understanding of the concepts of local/regional and systemic disease led to a diminished enthusiasm for bigger and bigger resections as the only answer for recurrent and/or unresectable cancers. In addition, the development of the capabilities for the use of radiation energy and chemical therapy for the control of cancer cell growth heralded the era of the multimodality approach to the management of many cancers. Nevertheless, these other modalities still served only an adjuvant role to the primary treatment of surgical resection. This relationship has evolved considerably in the last couple of decades, and with our current appreciation of the systemic nature of many cancers at the time of diagnosis, the surgeon has become an integral member of the multidisciplinary team who cares for the majority of patients with solid tumors. Thus the role of surgery and the surgeon in the management of patients with cancers involves a broad spectrum of 'conservative and radical' procedures tailored to the specific clinical setting and biology of the tumor involved. In particular, the stage of the tumor, the general state of health of the patient, the expected morbidity and mortality of the proposed procedure, and the probability for successful treatment of the tumor are all factors which impact on the decisions of whether to operate and what procedure to perform.

The remainder of this chapter will consider the roles of surgery in the screening, diagnosis, treatment and prevention of cancer.

SCREENING

The understanding of the epidemiology of many cancers has led to the identification of specific groups of patients who are at increased risk for developing certain cancers based on their genetic, demographic, and environmental associations. Examples of these include family history of breast and colon cancer, the associations of second primaries in patients with treated index cancers (e.g. breast and gynecologic malignancies), smoking related malignancies, and geographic clusters of certain cancers such as colorectal cancer in the United States. The surgeon is frequently the physician managing the follow-up care of these patients and thus is involved in screening for other tumors, counseling other family members regarding the need for surveillance, and performing specific surveillance examinations (e.g. breast exam with mammography, large bowel endoscopy, etc.) in those individuals with known increased risk.

DIAGNOSIS

Once a lesion has been identified, it is usually the role of the surgeon to provide adequate material to make a definitive diagnosis and allow for proper treatment planning. There are several ways to approach the acquisition of tissue for analysis including aspiration cytology (using a small needle to obtain single cells and clumps of cells for cytologic analysis), needle biopsy (using a large needle to obtain a core of tissue for histologic analysis), incisional biopsy, and excisional biopsy. The choice of method to be used needs to be carefully considered based upon the likely differential diagnoses, the amount of tissue required, the location of the lesion, and the potential forms of definitive treatment. For example, a cytologic specimen may be quite adequate for the identification of a breast cancer, but completely inadequate for the diagnosis of a lymphoma. An incisional biopsy is the appropriate approach for the diagnosis of a sarcoma, since an inadequate excisional biopsy may compromise the potential success of a later radical resection. An excisional biopsy with marking of the site and delineation of the resection margins is necessary for the evaluation of a mammographic abnormality to allow for the later potential use of primary radiation therapy without the necessity for rebiopsy before treatment. Finally, only a complete excision (i.e. total thyroid lobectomy) will allow for the differentiation of a follicular adenoma from a follicular carcinoma of the thyroid. In addition, the anatomic approach of the percutaneous needle puncture or the placement of a biopsy incision needs to be carefully planned to avoid injuring adjacent structures and to allow for subsequent excision of the 'contaminated' area at the time of the surgical resection.

Following the acquisition of tissue for a pathologic diagnosis, defining the stage of the disease is often required to complete the initial assessment and treatment plan. One example is the frequent need for staging laparotomy in the management of Hodgkins' disease, in which surgical exploration may change the clinical stage as often as 30% of the time. Another example is the need for axillary sampling to adequately stage patients with T1 and T2 breast cancers who have opted to receive primary radiation therapy to the breast. This information is necessary to determine the need for adjuvant hormonal and/or chemotherapy. For lung cancers, mediastinoscopy with nodal biopsy is an essential part of the determination of resectability for primary lung cancers.

TREATMENT

The role of surgery in the treatment of cancer patients takes many forms and is determined by the overall clinical status of the patient (age, general state of health, other disease processes), the specific biology of the tumor, and the stage of disease at the time of treatment. At times, the type and effects of other previous treatment modalities will also affect the need and form of surgical intervention.

Primary

Surgical resection remains the best form of curative treatment for most of the common solid tumors when they are diagnosed at an early stage (lung, breast, and colorectal). For these cancers, the improvement in overall survival has been due to a great extent to the ability to identify and thereby operate on patients at an earlier stage as a result of improved screening measures and increased patient/physician awareness. Unfortunately, the majority of cancers are still being diagnosed at a stage when surgical resection of the local disease is insufficient to result in a cure. Thus, much research effort and resources have been devoted to the development of effective multimodality treatment protocols aimed at improving the outcome in the majority of cancer patients. As examples, the addition of radiation and chemotherapy has decreased recurrence and improved survival in rectal cancer patients; recent studies of adjuvant levamisole and 5-FU have shown some improvement in the survival of certain colon cancer patients; and adjuvant chemotherapy has prolonged the disease free survival of many breast cancer patients.

In addition to this improvement in survival, the use of a multimodality approach to certain cancers has led to a decrease in the extent of the surgery required. The best examples of this are the use of radiation therapy in the treatment of Stage 1 breast cancer, which has allowed many patients to avoid mastectomy; and the combination of surgery and radiation therapy in the treatment of childhood rhabdomyosarcoma, which has greatly reduced the extent of resection and markedly improved survival. Finally, the use of combined therapy has resulted in the cure of certain tumors for which a single modality was unable to completely eradicate the gross tumor burden. The efficacy of such 'debulking or cytoreductive' procedures is best illustrated in the combination therapy approach to Burkitt's lymphoma and ovarian cancer. Another example is the use of intraoperative radiation therapy in combination with resection for locally recurrent rectal cancer. It is important to note, however, that cytoreductive surgery is rarely indicated in those settings where no effective chemotherapy or radiation therapy is available. Nevertheless, more effective chemotherapy, radiotherapy, and immunotherapy will hopefully extend the indications for this multimodality approach.

Metastases

The role of surgical resection in the treatment of metastatic disease is becoming a better defined and more often applied therapy, especially for tumors which are poorly responsive to other modalities. As a general principle, these metastatic sites need to be solitary or at least focally clustered (e.g. in a single lobe of the liver) for this approach to be effective, and unfortunately this presentation is uncommon. Nevertheless, resectable pulmonary metastases from soft tissue and bony sarcomas can be cured with surgery in up to 30% of patients. Similarly, resection of localized lung and liver metastases from colorectal cancers will cure 25% of these patients. This is certainly superior to the results of nonsurgical treatment of these lesions. Finally, solitary brain metastases should be evaluated for resection based on the primary tumor (e.g. colon vs. breast) and the morbidity associated with the resection.

Palliation

The surgeon is often asked to consider methods for symptomatic relief, improvement of functional status or to manage complications resulting from other treatment modalities in patients who are not likely to be cured of their cancer. Partial resections or intestinal bypasses for gastrointestinal obstruction, removal of a large symptomatic breast cancer in a patient with widespread metastases, placement of a gastrostomy drainage or feeding tube, and operative neurolysis for pain relief are all examples in which the potential for symptomatic relief and improvement in functional status need to be weighed against the predicted mortality and morbidity of the surgery. In addition, patients undergoing rigorous chemotherapy and radiation therapy not uncommonly develop emergent complications such as gastrointestinal hemorrhage or perforations, sepsis from abscess formation, etc. Once again, the approach to the management of these complications needs to be individualized to the clinical setting with regard to the type of tumor, stage of disease, potential efficacy of therapy, and the wishes of the patient.

Reconstruction

Advances in the field of plastic and reconstructive surgery, especially with the advent of microvascular surgery and tissue transfer techniques, has led to the ability to safely and reasonably perform more extensive resections, and also to modify and decrease the functional and cosmetic morbidity associated with some more traditional surgical procedures. A good example of the latter situation is the ability to perform simultaneous breast reconstruction at the time of mastectomy. This has provided an excellent option for patients who are either unable or unwilling to undergo breast preservation with radiation therapy. The functional morbidity and disfigurement which were the frequent sequelae of major resections and/ or high dose radiation therapy for head and neck cancers have been greatly diminished by the use of microvascular composite graft transfers. In addition, the functional disability of extremities can be improved through the use of muscle transfers, homologous bone grafts, and implantable prosthetics.

PREVENTION

As our understanding of tumorogenesis expands and our ability to recognize premalignant lesions improves, the role for surgery in the prevention of cancers will continue to increase. The removal of sporadic adenomatous colorectal polyps with either surgical or endoscopic polypectomy will certainly reduce the incidence of colorectal cancer to some extent. We know that patients with familial polyposis coli have nearly a 100% incidence of developing carcinoma and patients with long standing ulcerative colitis who develop areas of dysplasia have a >50% incidence of developing carcinoma. Prophylactic proctocolectomy in these patients will prevent these cancers. Patients with noninvasive intraductal carcinoma of the breast have a 70% probability of developing ipsilateral invasive breast cancer. Women with a mother and sister who have had premenopausal breast cancer have more than a 50% chance of developing breast cancer. Certainly, prophylactic mastectomy with or without reconstruction is an important option to consider in these cases. Patients with MEN II syndrome and familial C-cell hyperplasia should be screened with pentagastrin stimulated serum calcitonin tests in order to identify those patients who will need thyroidectomy to prevent medullary carcinoma of the thyroid. These are some examples of situations in which surgical removal of a target organ will prevent cancer development in certain high risk individuals.

Thus we see that surgery and the surgical oncologist play an integral although somewhat modified role in the multidisciplinary approach to the care of patients with cancer. Close interaction and collaboration between these multiple oncologic specialists in the management of patients and the development and conduct of basic and clinical research are essential to insure the continued improvement in the treatment of patients with cancer.

Chapter 9

Radiation Oncology

Radiation oncology is a distinct specialty that deals with the use of radiation in the treatment of malignancy. There are very few indications for the utilization of radiation in benign diseases. Radiation can be used to treat virtually all cancers in all age groups in all primary sites. It can used as a primary treatment modality with curative intent, especially in small, relatively localized cancers. Examples include irradiation for localized breast cancer or for carcinoma of the larynx. Radiation can also be used with a palliative intent to treat locally advanced cancers or metastatic cancers once they have caused symptoms. Radiation can also be used in combined modality programs added to either chemotherapy and/or surgery. It can also be used as an adjuvant to surgery. Many newer strategies for cancer management are being devised that use radiation in nonconventional ways to try to enhance tumor cell kill while sparing normal tissue.

THE FIELD OF RADIATION ONCOLOGY

The administration of ionizing radiation to patients is only one part of the broad specialty of radiation oncology. Pre-treatment definition of the extent of a cancer, evaluation of patients for irradiation, care during irradiation, and post-treatment care and follow up examinations are essential to good cancer management which translates into good patient care. This specialty demands an in-depth knowledge of the origin and clinical evolution of cancer as well as the efficacy of alternate methods of treatment, and indepth background in both the physics and radiobiology of ionizing radiation is critical to its proper use in the clinical management of cancer. Once the clinical distribution (stage), clinical evolution, and growth characteristics of cancer are understood and the radiation tolerances of the associated normal tissues are appreciated, the techniques of irradiating the volume of interest are problems of geometry, physics, and mechanics. The machinery necessary to deliver proper therapeutic radiation are very large and complicated. Radiation oncology departments are usually located within the basement of a facility to take advantage of natural shielding from the ground. The size and complexity of the technology necessary to deliver modern radiation treatments dwarfs virtually every other technology within a hospital. Many "free standing" facilities have developed throughout this country, and most will offer guided tours upon request.

It is important to understand the difference between a radiation oncologist and a general radiologist. Radiation oncology uses high energy x-rays to kill malignant tissue. This is a separate specialty that requires 4 years of training plus 1 or 2 fellowship years. A general radiologist uses low energy radiation to visualize anatomy. This distinct specialty also requires approximately 5 years of training. Low energy radiation will allow adequate contrast between various tissue densities, and its use provides essential information for the radiation oncologist as well as medical oncologist and surgeon. Proximity to a well equipped radiology department is essential for good cancer management.

There are many specific terms utilized by the experts in this modality. Terms such as rad, ret, rem, Roentgen, centigray (cGy), portal, teletherapy, brachytherapy, shielding, half life, etc. are all specific to the modality. If there is ever a question regarding the meaning of these terms or how they relate to a cancer patient's care, a phone call to the radiation oncologist in charge of a particular patient can be used for clarification. All too often, physicians in unrelated medical specialties will overlook the major role that the radiation oncologist plays in the treatment of cancer. This is often because of lack of detailed knowledge of the modality and can be simply resolved by either a phone call or a visit with the radiation oncologist.

Most of the radiation oncologist's time is in direct patient management. This involves the supervision and coordination of many patients under treatment at any one time. The close individual attention requires that the radiation oncologist spend the predominant portion of time near the treatment machines. Many of the technical details require individual attention and this can most efficiently be rendered through the direct attention of the radiation oncologist. The usual patient load for a radiation oncologist would be 15 to 25 patients under treatment at any one time.

"Curative" radiation can be delivered to as many as 50% of patients who are referred to a radiation oncologist. Radiation can be delivered alone or with surgery either pre-operatively, post-operativel, or both. It can also be delivered during surgery (intraoperative radiation) once the cancer has been properly exposed. Radiation can be delivered with chemotherapy, immunotherapy, or combined in a true multimodality approach. The cancers commonly treated for cure with primary radiation include early breast cancer, Hodgkin's disease and other lymphomas, cancers of the cervix and endometrium, germ cell tumors in both the testes and ovary, prostate cancer, most head and neck cancers, early cancer of the lung and esophagus, localized cancers of the rectum and anal canal, soft tissue sarcomas, pediatric cancers, brain tumors, and nonmelanomatous skin cancers. Radiation is even integrated into the treatment of certain leukemias, especially in the setting of bone marrow transplantation.

Palliative irradiation offers relief of symptoms or the prevention of serious consequences, for example, to relieve pain from bone metastases. A patient would be treated in the area causing pain usually over the course of 2 to 3 weeks. The radiation typically relieves the pain during the second week of administration and the pain usually continues to improve for 2 to 4 weeks beyond the treatment time. Other examples of palliation would be the treatment of brain and spinal cord metastases from virtually any primary site. The brain and spinal cord are quite radioresistant, allowing a significant therapeutic advantage. Other palliative situations would include bleeding (e.g. hemoptysis from lung cancer or uterine bleeding from cervical cancer).

Patients characteristically have treatments delivered on a daily basis throughout a standard work week. A course of radiation that is to be delivered with curative intent may take 6 to 8 weeks. The intention is to deliver a certain relative dose of radiation over a certain relative period of time. Details such as field size, dose rate, and location of the target volume would dictate the most appropriate treatment schedule. Radiation treatments are delivered in units called "fractions" that are usually delivered once per day. Alternate treatment fractionation schedules are being investigated clinically and the utility may grow as clinical trials mature. A palliative course of radiation may involve 10 to 15 fractions administered over 2 to 3 weeks, once again on a daily basis 5 days a week. In this setting, the goals of treatment must be conveyed to the patient so that a realistic expectation can be maintained. A typical treatment span of time on any one day may be 15 to 20 minutes. The majority of treatments are given to patients on an outpatient basis. A patient would come in, receive their treatment and then go home. They would not be radioactive and they would otherwise be able to conduct their activities normally.

The radiation oncologist must supervise the details of treatment, management of side effects, and provision of emotional support. Modification of treatment volumes depend upon both the patient and tumor response to that treatment. While many specific details regarding dose and indications for treatment are important, *individualization* of treatment is the key to success in any given patient's cancer management. Follow-up examinations are also essential. For example, a typical follow-up schedule for a patient with Hodgkin's disease or some other lymphoma may be rather frequent in the period immediately following treatment since 85% of recurrences occur within 2 years. Therefore, the follow-up visits are more intense during that period of time. Ninety per cent of head and neck cancers will recur within the first 2 years, and follow-up schedules are constructed accordingly. Patients need to be followed for the longer term as well to see if new primaries occur or to observe for any potential long term side effects from treatment. Breast and prostate cancers have a much more protracted natural history, and follow-up for these malignancies may go on for more than 20 years. It is imperative to watch for signs of any residual, recurrent, or metastatic disease so that early intervention can be facilitated. It is extremely important to recognize and treat long term side effects of radiation.

A premium must be placed upon caring for the patient's emotional and symptomatic needs. There also needs to be close cooperation with other cancer specialists enabling the integration of multiple therapeutic modalities.

BRIEF REVIEW OF RADIOBIOLOGY

Radiation is a nonspecific cytotoxic agent. It can kill any cell or tissue if given in a high enough dose. The killing involves a physical interaction of high energy interactions between molecules. The goal of treatment is to kill all the malignant cells without producing "too much" damage to the normal cells around these malignant ones. The "art" is to aim the beam of radiation exactly where you want it, maximizing the effects on the tumor while minimizing the effects on normal tissue.

A major biological factor in the utilization of radiation is that multiple "sublethal" doses of radiation are given over a defined period of time. It takes normal tissue approximately 4 hours to *repair* any radiation damage whereas malignant tissue takes a much longer period of time for this repair. Over a course of treatment, multiple sublethal events occur during this period of time and the malignant tissue cannot recover from this injury but normal tissue can repair this damage. This is how a non-specific killing agent such as ionizing radiation can be rendered specific for malignancy.

Radiation sensitivity of cells depends upon the phase of their reproductive cycle and on the number of chromosomes in their nucleus. The cell is most sensitive during the phase of mitosis and least sensitive during the phase of meiosis. Radiation kills cells, stimulating other cells to divide, causing *repopulation* within the tumor and *redistribution* within the cell cycle.

Free radical interactions with DNA can cause cross linkages that will alter the genetic message for that portion of DNA. If the damage is not repaired the cell may lose critical protein synthesis functions and this will ultimately result in cell death. If cells are dormant from a protein synthetic standpoint, for example slowly dividing, the damage may not be expressed until the cells attempt mitosis. Radiation does not "vaporize" malignant tissue, but does alter the ability of a given cell to divide. Once this cell goes through the cycle and is unable to divide, normal body mechanisms take over with removal of that dead cell. Oxygen is the ultimate radiation sensitizer, and cell kill from radiation allows for *reoxygenation* facilitating more cytotoxicity.

The four R's of radiation are thus: repair, repopulation, redistribution, and reoxygenation.

The tolerance to radiation for normal tissue in any anatomical location is well defined. The task of the radiation oncologist is to administer a quality of radiation sufficient to kill the malignancy while minimizing any substantial damage to normal tissue. In certain areas, such as an extremity, this may be relatively simple. The tolerance to external radiation of bone, soft tissue, and skin, as well as major blood vessels is quite high. In other locations such as the upper abdomen, normal tissue will substantially limit the amount of radiation that can be administered. The small intestine, large intestine, liver, pancreas, and stomach as well as kidney are much more sensitive to radiation than are cancers that occur in that area.

The process of deciding exactly how to give a certain prescribed dose to a certain area is called treatment planning. The first step is simulation. A machine called a simulator allows the radiation oncologist to visualize the tumor in three dimensions. Data from the CAT scan or other x-ray procedures are analyzed by a computer program, and a plan to maximize the dose to the tumor and minimize the dose to the surrounding normal tissues is generated. Once the plan is implemented, careful checks on the energy and "scatter" of the beam must be done. The fields must be reproducible on a daily basis.

The types of radiation are listed below:

Electromagnetic—   x-rays
                   gamma rays
Particulate—   electrons (beta particles)
                   protons
                   neutrons
                   alpha particles
                   pi mesons

Electromagnetic radiation (also called photons) has no charge and no mass x-rays are produced by man-made machines in which an electron is accelerated in a charged field to strike a target (usually tungston or gold) producing photons of specific energies. The machine is called a linear accelerator. If no target is present, an "electron beam" can be produced. The other type of electromagnetic radiation, called gamma rays (which are identical to x-rays or photons except for the source) are produced by natural decay of radioactive isotopes like cobalt-60. Different sources of radiation may have different energies and different "depths" into tissue where their energy will be dissipated.

Particulate radiation (other than x-rays mentioned above) can be produced by certain radioisotopes that can be used as implants or "tagged" to certain monoclonal antibodies. This type of radiation is also produced at certain large research facilities like Los Alamos in New Mexico.

The biologic effects observed for one type of radiation may be produced by virtually any other type of irradiation. None of these biological effects produced by radiation are unique solely to radiation, but are at least superficially indistinguishable from effects produced by other agents. The amount of energy required to produce biological effects is extremely small. We are all exposed to low levels of radiation, and in the aggregate, this exposure causes thousands of cancer cases each year. One must make a distinction between the physical event of receiving radiation and the biologic events that will result in tumor shrinkage within the treatment field. Radiation is associated with mutation, carcinogenesis, and teratogenesis. There is a hierarchy of cell sensitivity to radiation. The most sensitive cells are the bone marrow stem cells, germ cells, and intestinal epithelium. Less sensitive cells include those of epidermal origin, vascular, thyroid, and lung epithelium. The least sensitive cells are those of muscle, bone, cartilage, and nervous system tissue.

Certain cancers are radioresistant. This is always a relative term, since some tumors that are radioresistant may be radiocurable, while some tumors that are radiosensitive (e.g. leukemias) are not radiocurable. Primary central nervous system cancers are one example of a radioresistant tumor. Since radioresistance is a relative term, strategies have been devised to treat CNS cancers with very high doses of localized radiation through neurosurgical implantation techniques for the delivery of high dose radiation via isotopes such as iridium.

Side effects of radiation are related to dose, fields, and areas or organs being treated. Nausea may be treated with antiemetics, diarrhea with antispasmodics, and mucositis with soothing topical preparations like Benadryl-Maalox solutions. Long term side effects include those related to fibrosis of the organ treated, e.g. pulmonary fibrosis. Second malignancies can occur but they are relatively rare.

FUTURE PROSPECTS

There is an ongoing quest to develop better means for more early detection of malignancy and for improving therapeutic strategies. These would include the combination of chemotherapeutic agents integrated specifically into the irradiation sequence; hyperfractionation, or the delivery of more than one radiation treatment per day; photodynamic therapy, which is the use of "light" reactive agents that will enhance the effect of radiation on malignant tissues; hyperthermia, or the delivery of heat to a tumor volume to specifically kill malignant cells and enhance the effects of radiation; radiation sensitizers, or the use of chemicals that will mimic the effects of oxygen in the centers of cancers where hypoxia is present; particle therapy, or the use of alpha particles, protons or neutrons to treat cancer; intraoperative irradiation; radiolabeled monoclonal antibodies; brachytherapy; and the use of implants.

Combined modality therapy is the use of chemotherapeutic agents integrated specifically within the irradiation sequence. Drugs can be administered before, during, or after the radiation sequence. The intent is to maximize tumor cell kill and minimize side effects. Certain chemotherapeutic agents can also enhance the effect of radiation if given in a specifically timed manner. Particular attention must be paid to the dose of the chemotherapeutic agent used as well as its timing in relation to the administration of radiation. This has become a popular strategy for the treatment of locally advanced head and neck cancers. The drugs currently being used with radiation include cisplatin or its analogs, 5-fluorouracil, and mitomycin C. It is important to try to minimize the side effects of each agent and maximize the tumor cell kill.

Altered fractionation tries to take advantage of the simple concept that normal tissue can repair radiation damage on a molecular level within 3 to 4 hours post treatment. Therefore, a dose given every 6 hours could enhance tumor cell kill and not exacerbate normal tissue injury. This strategy is particularly attractive in the treatment of locally advanced but unresectable lung cancers. From a biologic standpoint if normal tissue damage can be minimized, total doses of radiation could be carried to higher levels and this should improve local tumor control. Multi-institutional cooperative groups such as the Radiation Therapy Oncology Group (RTOG), Cancer and Acute Leukemia Group B (CALGB), and Pediatric Oncology Group (POG) are actively investigating this approach.

Photodynamic therapy has gained a great deal of interest in the past several years. This utilizes agents that are taken up by a cell and activated with the delivery of specific wavelengths of light. Breakdown products of normal red blood cells (called hematoporphyrin derivatives) have been utilized. These concentrate in cancer cells and when certain wavelenths of ultraviolet light are administered, the cells can be killed specifically while sparing normal tissue.

Hyperthermia is a treatment of cancer that has been of experimental interest for the past 15 years. Although there has been a long history of the use of heat to treat cancers, within the mid 1960's more fundamental work was undertaken to develop heat as another cancer therapy. Heat alone can kill malignant cells, and the temperature necessary for this cell killing effect is 42.5 to 45° centigrade (about the temperature of a hot bath). If a tumor volume can be raised to this temperature, the preferential destruction of malignant tissue will occur. Hyperthermia has been used with radiation as a potentiating agent. Hyperthermia may be particularly useful in areas of low oxygen tension (i.e. the hypoxic, necrotic centers of tumors). Certain devices have been developed which can deliver heat to a variety of tumor sites very specifically. The engineering to develop devices that will deliver specific temperatures throughout a tumor volume is very difficult but very exciting. The goal is to specifically heat only the tumor without heating normal tissue. Heat delivered by itself in the 40° centigrade temperature range can increase blood flow to those tissues being irradiated. If carried to a slightly higher temperature of 41.5 to 42° centigrade, specific cyotoxicity for malignant tissue can occur. Raising this temperature to 42.5 to 43° centigrade can cause additional tumor cell kill, especially at low pH and in tumor cell compartments that are going through synthetic (or S) phase. Above 43° centigrade, vascular destruction occurs within tumor tissue and above 46° centigrade vascular destruction can occur even within normal tissue. These effects of heating on malignant tissue have been extensively evaluated in the laboratory. Clinical trials to take advantage of the cytotoxic potential of heat and radiation are currently under way. While heat by itself is a relatively inefficient cytotoxic agent, it can be very efficient if combined with radiation (and, it appears, with certain chemotherapeutic agents). The effects of hyperthermia properly relate more to a cell membrane phenomenon than a nuclear phenomenon as does radiation. In addition, malignant tissue has an altered vasculature that is much more sensitive to this modality than is normal tissue. An entire literature has developed about the use of hyperthermia in cancer management, and specific details can be obtained from the radiation oncologist.

Radiation sensitizers are chemicals that when present in a tumor can enhance the effect of radiation. They are substances that diffuse into the poorly oxygenated centers of tumor masses. Most of the radiation sensitizers are chemicals that have specific side effects. The compounds used to date include metronidazole, misonidazole, and a new compound called SR-2508. Although the enhancement of radiation killing of tumor cells is seen in animals and in vitro, clinical trials have shown no enhanced effects.

Certain chemotherapeutic agents also enhance the effects of radiation when given in a very specific time-dose related sequence. The platinum compounds have undergone extensive clinical trials in this regard. These agents can also be utilized for their direct therapeutic effect. Other agents include 5-fluorouracil, mitomycin C, and the nitrosoureas (especially BCNU).

Particle beam therapy involves the use of protons or neutrons or heavier particles (e.g. alpha particles) for the treatment of cancers. Each of these has a very specific absorption pattern of their energy in tissue. Neutron beam therapy provides much more densely ionizing radiation and has 10 times the destructive capability of photon beam or electron therapy. Proton beam therapy deals with the concept of a "Bragg" peak. There is a specific point at which almost all of the energy is released in a very short area, sparing the tissue passed through on entry. This may be useful to treat such tumors as pituitary tumors, with "all" the energy going to a specific place. Ongoing physics work has been done to manipulate this "Bragg" peak to a therapeutic advantage. Very few facilities have the abilities to treat with neutron or proton beams.

Another new advance is intraoperative irradiation. This is conceptually a very simple procedure in which the radiation is delivered during the operative procedure with actual physical withdrawal of normal tissue from the radiation field. To coordinate the delivery of radiation with an open surgical wound is a cumbersome task. Many institutions in this country utilize a linear accelerator to deliver an electron beam during an intraoperative procedure. Other institutions have placed a low energy x-ray machine in an operating room that can be used much more efficiently during the surgical procedure. Single large doses of radiation have been given and their subsequent biological effects studied. Some institutions have also devised systems to deliver hyperthermia directly during an operative procedure.

A new modality to target malignant tissue is that of radiolabeled monoclonal antibodies. The prototype for this treatment approach is thyroid cancer. For papillary and mixed papillary-follicular carcinomas of the thyroid, the tendency of this tissue to take up iodine is exploited. If an isotope of iodine is administered, it will go directly to the tumor site, deliver its radiation, and spare normal surrounding tissue. Over the past 5 to 10 years, the development of monoclonal antibodies for delivery of cancer toxins has been actively investigated. Various isotopes have been evalu-

ated, including I-125 and yttrium-90. A major effort to quantita
doses delivered to these tumor volumes over time by this "Trojan hor
therapy is under way. The specificity of the antibody for malignant tissue
is very important. If they target normal tissue as well, there may be no
therapeutic advantage.

Finally, the ability to place radioactive material within a tumor volume
has also undergone a resurgence of interest. Brachytherapy, derived from
Greek, means "short range" therapy. If one places catheters throughout
a tumor volume in a specific geometrical array, then radioactive material
(and also hyperthermia) can be delivered through these conduits. A good
example would be the implantation into brain tumors of such catheters.
These are very difficult tumors to control with external beam radiation,
surgery, or chemotherapy alone or in combination. However, with ste-
reotactic technique and more modern neurosurgical abilities, catheters
can be placed within a relatively well defined tumor volume. Through
these catheters, various therapeutic agents can be administered. Intense
effort is now under way to analyze these approaches in various clinical
trials. Irradiating the tumor from the inside outward as this does has a
strong conceptual attraction. Delivery of hyperthermia or chemotherapy
by this approach is also possible.

Those wishing to learn further details about the use of radiation against
cancer should consult *Therapeutic Radiology for the House Officer* by
Lawrence R. Coria, M.D., and David J. Moylan, M.D., published by Williams & Wilkins, Baltimore/London.

Chapter 10

ancer Chemotherapy

Perhaps as important as the knowledge of various drugs' uses and toxicities is an appreciation of the philosophic rationale for a given chemotherapeutic effort. A legitimate attempt at curative therapy may justify considerable toxicity and risk, especially in younger or more durable patients. Palliative treatment (to relieve symptoms) in order to prolong survival may be appropriate even if it entails moderate morbidity; palliative treatment to relieve symptoms but not increase survival ideally should have little toxicity. Patients who are expected to have brief survival due to end-stage tumor involvement or refractory disease merit supportive care, and an option not to treat at all with chemotherapy should be strongly considered. It is essential that the treating physician and the patient both understand the goals and limitations of treatment.

In considering general tumor types where chemotherapy may or may not be successful, a number of accepted categories exist. A partial list of the more common malignancies is as follows:

1. Cure or prolonged survival expected:
   a. Hodgkin's disease
   b. Large cell non-Hodgkin's lymphoma
   c. Testicular carcinoma
   d. Childhood leukemia and lymphoma

2. Some survival benefit expected:
   a. Breast carcinoma
   b. Ovarian carcinoma
   c. Small cell carcinoma of lung
   d. Non-Hodgkin's lymphoma
   e. Multiple myeloma

3. Palliation expected:
   a. Prostate carcinoma
   b. Bladder carcinoma
   c. Endometrial carcinoma
   d. Head and neck carcinoma

4. Palliation possible:
   a. Non-small cell lung carcinoma
   b. Colorectal carcinoma
   c. Soft tissue sarcomas
   d. Melanoma

A unique situation in which chemotherapy is increasingly employed is that of *adjuvant* treatment. Classically this pertains to a situation where a primary tumor has been grossly eradicated with surgery or radiation, yet judging from historical data, a predictably common frequency of relapse exists due to subclinical micrometastases. Despite the fact that an immediate tumor response cannot be measured (providing some type of tumor marker is not present) and the knowledge that some patients may in fact have no residual malignancy, chemotherapy with known active agents may be given for a predetermined period of time. Major advantages with this approach include theoretically low numbers of viable tumor cells and likely a small percentage of resistant cells. Adjuvant chemotherapy is generally administered in the setting of an investigational protocol, or when a proven benefit has been demonstrated by such studies.

CHEMOTHERAPY

The most frequent therapeutic modality utilized to control or reduce the burden of systemic malignancy is cytotoxic chemotherapy. From initial efforts with single agent treatments to the current era of multiple drug (standard or investigational) regimens, a formidable inventory of agents with their attendant actions and toxicities now exists. An understanding of each agent, whether used alone or in concert with others, is fundamental to the practice and evolution of clinical oncology.

One helpful concept relating cellular behavior and the effects of chemotherapy is the "cell cycle" (Fig. 10.1). Following mitosis (M), a typical cell spends a variable period of time in the first gap phase (G1), where

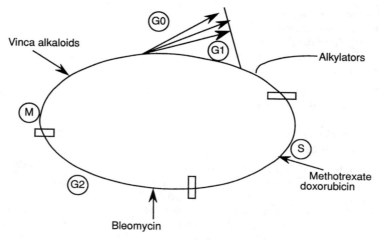

Figure 10.1   The Cell Cycle

DNA repair may take place, and synthesis of RNA and protein ensue. From G1 a cell may enter a prolonged resting phase (Go) of variable duration, prior to reentering the cycle. At the completion of G1, a phase of DNA synthesis (S) occurs. A second gap phase (G2), where RNA and protein synthesis continues, then brings the cell to the verge of mitosis and subsequent cell division.

M phase: mitosis; usually lasts 30–90 minutes. G_1 phase: most variable phase, from brief to prolonged (due to timing of G_0)—late G_1 associated with an increase in DNA replicative enzymes. G_0 phase: resting phase—may last months. S phase: DNA synthesis with increased activity of replicative DNA synthesis with increased activity of replicative enzymes, e.g. DNA polynerase, thymidine kinase, and dihydrofolate reductase. Lasts 8–30 hrs. G2 phase: second gap; usually 1–2 hrs. long. Representative examples of certain chemotherapy drugs are shown, associated with phases where they exert a major effect.

Chemotherapy agents typically exert their influence in certain phases of the cell cycle. Antimetabolites, such as methotrexate, are phase specific for the S phase, whereas bleomycin and daunorubicin are most effective in G2. The vinca alkaloids, vincristine and vinblastine, are particularly active during mitosis. Certain agents (e.g. 5-fluorouracil and cyclophosphamide) are toxic to both resting cells and cells that are actively proceeding through the cycle, though the active cells are more sensitive; cis-diamminedichloroplatinum (C-DDP) and the nitrosoureas are equally toxic to both resting and cycling cells.

Both normal cells and cancer cells have their own characteristic cell cycles, occasionally with considerable similarities. Rapidly growing normal tissues such as bone marrow, gastrointestinal mucosa, and hair follicles may have a higher percentage of cells actively in cycle compared to many malignancies. Even in this setting, however, malignant cells may accumulate faster than their normal tissue counterparts; a failure to mature in a timely fashion and/or an abnormally prolonged life span allow this to happen. Both normal and malignant cell populations may undergo early exponential growth; normal cells will reach a steady state where renewal and cell loss are balanced, but malignant cell populations will continue to expand, finally reaching such a volume that the growth rate necessarily slows down. Indeed, the late-occurring increase in doubling time of an expanding tumor reflects a decrease in growth fraction and more cell loss (likely due to an inevitably inefficient vascular and nutrient supply).

A tumor can be detected when it is as small as 1 cm^3, which corresponds to approximately 10^9 cells or 30 doublings (most tumors double in 10–165 days). A 1-kg mass (considered to be a lethal amount of malignancy in humans) represents 10^{12} cells and is equivalent to 40 doublings. Thus, by the time of detection, a malignancy is quite far along (3/4) in its natural history. Based on observations made by Skipper and Schabel, it is generally accepted that a given chemotherapy agent will kill a fixed percentage of cells in a given tumor; this has been designated the concept of "log kill." If a drug kills 99.9% of cells with one treatment, it will reduce a tumor of 10^{10} cells to 10^7; similarly, a tumor with 10^7 cells (at which point it likely may be undetectable) will decrease to 10^4. To potentially effect a cure in this setting, multiple treatments will be required.

If human malignancies were comprised of homogeneous cell populations uniformly sensitive to chemotherapy agents, the treatment of metastatic tumors would often be successful. Unfortunately, this is not the case. Malignancies are usually heterogeneous and tend to be even more so at high volumes. In addition, at high tumor volumes a greater percentage of cells may be resting, a state relatively insensitive to many chemotherapy agents. A resting cell partially damaged by chemotherapy may be able to repair itself before cell division when it would be most vulnerable to prior damage.

Random genetic changes occur in malignant cells, some of which may confer resistance to chemotherapy drugs—the larger the tumor cell population, the more likely there will be resistant clones. Baseline mutation rates will vary from tumor to tumor, and cells multiply resistant to agents may evolve in situations where mutation rates are high.

Cell inactivity and mutational events are only two reasons why cells may become temporarily resistant to chemotherapeutic agents. Certain malignancies may be sensitive to only a small number of drugs, which may be effective in only certain phases of the cell cycle, thus precluding a broad effect. Physiologic sanctuaries (CSF, testicles) may provide a haven for viable malignant cells where drugs cannot reach them in appropriate amounts.

A more permanent resistance may evolve with changes in the drug transport mechanisms of malignant cells, as those cells with less drug uptake or facilitated efflux maintain a growth advantage. Tumor cells may also develop more efficient metabolic pathways, resulting in a quicker breakdown of active drugs. An increase in DNA repair capabilities or an increase in drug binding sites leading to inactivation may also confer resistance. Poor tumor vascularity may also decrease drug delivery to cells. Certain tumor cells may even develop a curious property called "pleiotropic drug resistance," where resistance to one chemotherapy agent may be associated with de novo resistance to other agents to which the tumor cell has not been exposed. In summary, early treatment of a tumor when its volume is small may be most successful since the growth rate is high and resistance is less likely.

Principles in Chemotherapy Planning

There are a number of common principles employed in developing chemotherapy strategies. Some of the most important concepts are as follows:

1. Selection of individual agents should be based on demonstrated specific anti-tumor activity; especially valuable are those agents which can produce complete remissions.

2. Combination chemotherapy programs with multiple effective agents are generally more successful than single agent treatments. In certain malignancies that are unlikely to be cured (e.g. indolent lymphomas), however, single agent treatment may easily induce a remission with less toxicity.

3. Chemotherapy combinations ideally will include agents with different modes of action or with known anti-tumor synergism.

4. The expected toxicities of each agent in a program ideally will not overlap.

5. Maximum doses and optimal scheduling should be employed, with the shortest possible interval between treatments (allowing normal tissues to recover).

6. Avoid dose lowering or delaying tactics to alleviate mild to moderate toxicity, since major deviations in anti-tumor activity may ensue. Consider specific supportive measures to address toxicities where appropriate (e.g. antiemetics, dietary supplementation, support groups, etc.)

7. Assess response data after one or two cycles of treatment since, in the great majority of malignancies, a response should materialize prior to the third cycle (usually by 6–8 weeks after the beginning of treatment). One notable exception is breast carcinoma, which may take longer to respond. No response after two cycles generally predicts little, if any, therapeutic benefit, and progression at any time is a sufficient reason to stop a current regimen.

8. In the event of a true response, most clinicians consider a total of 6–12 cycles of chemotherapy to achieve optimal anti-tumor effect.

Specific Chemotherapy Agents

The following section reviews specific uses and toxicities of various commonly used chemotherapeutic medications. One should keep in mind that virtually all cytotoxic agents are potentially carcinogenic; just as they may damage malignant cells in a beneficial manner, instances of secondary malignancies evolving from sublethally damaged normal tissues do exist. Fortunately, secondary malignancies are relatively rare.

BCNU
(Carmustine; BiCNU®)

Physical Properties and Mechanisms

One of a class of alkylators (agents that substitute a hydrocarbon radical for a hydrogen atom in a cyclic compound) called nitrosoureas.

Alkylates DNA and RNA; not cross-resistant with other alkylators.

May also inhibit enzyme processes by carbamylation of amino acids in proteins.

High lipid solubility allowing effective traversing of blood-brain barrier.

60–70% of drug excreted in urine over 96 hours.

Dosage:

150–200 mg/m^2 IV every 6 weeks (administration in less than 1 hour may result in local burning at IV site or flushing).

Indications:

Brain tumors, myeloma, lymphomas

Toxicities:

Bone Marrow—effects on marrow may be delayed as long as 6 weeks (usual nadir 4–6 weeks) and effects are cumulative—thrombocytopenia may be particularly severe.

Pulmonary Fibrosis—likely dose related, especially if dose greater than 1400 mg/m^2—rarely fatal.

Gastrointestinal—nausea, vomiting common (risk period usually lasts 4–6 hr.).

Hepatotoxicity—mild, usually reversible.

Renal Failure—uncommon; usually with higher cumulative doses.

Dermatologic—external irritant.

Precautions:

Monitor blood counts prior to each cycle and be sure adequate levels of WBC and platelets are maintained.

Check pulmonary function tests if symptomatic or with high cumulative doses (parameters ≤ 70% of normal are worrisome).

BLEOMYCIN
(Blenoxane®)

Physical Properties and Mechanisms:

Mixture of cytotoxic antibiotics isolated from a strain of *Streptomyces.*

Measured in units, not milligrams.

Non specific inhibitor of DNA synthesis, and to a lesser degree, RNA and protein synthesis.

Dosage:

Test dose: 2 units or less for 1–2 doses to assess for idiosyncratic response.

Usual dose: 0.25–0.5 units/kg IV, IM or SQ weekly or less frequently (avoid greater than 400 units if possible).

Indications:

Head and neck carcinomas, lymphomas (Hodgkin's and non-Hodgkin's), testicular carcinoma.

Toxicities:

Pulmonary—up to 10% may get pneumonitis which can progress to fibrosis. More common if age greater than 70 or total dose greater than 400 u. Dyspnea earliest symptom, diffusion capacity (D_LCO) drop of greater than or equal to 30% compared to pretreatment value is reason to stop.

Dermatologic—up to 50% may develop varying degrees of rash, vesiculation, hyperpigmentation, tenderness, nail changes, stomatitis.

Idiosyncratic Reactions—1%, similar to anaphylaxis; fever, chills, wheezing, hypotension (treatment is symptomatic).

Precautions:

Patients previously treated with bleomycin are at greater risk of developing pulmonary toxicity with oxygen therapy (at high F_IO_2's) during surgery (anesthesiologists should be forewarned).

CARBOPLATIN
(Paraplatin®)

Physical Properties and Mechanisms:

Like cis-diamminedichloroplatinum (C-DDP), produces interstrand DNA crosslinks.

Activity cell cycle nonspecific.

Renal excretion major route.

Dosage:

As single agent, 360 mg/m² over 15–30 minutes every 4 weeks (if creatinine clearance 41–59 ml/min, 250 mg/m²; if 16–40 ml/min, 200 mg/m²).

Indications:

Ovarian carcinoma, lung carcinomas (may eventually have same spectrum of activity as C-DDP).

Toxicities:

Bone marrow suppression—usually moderate; mean nadir about day 21-hemoglobin below 11 gm% common.

Renal—limited, yet may be increased with concomitant aminoglycoside use.

Gastrointestinal—nausea/vomiting common though usually doesn't last more than 24 hours. Also abdominal pain, diarrhea, constipation.

Neurologic—limited (worsens in 30% of patients with neurotoxicity from C-DDP).

Allergic Reaction—1–2% (symptomatic treatment).

Hepatic—mild LFT changes (usually at greater than or equal to $4 \times$ recommended doses).

Electrolyte—may see Na^+, K^+, Ca^{++}, Mg^{++} lowering.

Dermatologic—alopecia rare.

Precautions:

Aluminum needles may precipitate platinum and thus decrease its potency.

Bone Marrow Suppression more severe if prior exposure to chemotherapy, or with renal dysfunction.

Vigorous hydration unnecessary.

CHLORAMBUCIL
(Leukeran ®)

Physical Properties and Mechanisms:

Like melphalan, a bifunctional alkylator rapidly and well absorbed from GI tract. Metabolized quickly in liver; plasma protein bound.

Dosage:

0.1–0.2 mg/kg per day for 3–6 week period followed by reduction to a maintenance dose (0.03–0.1 mg/kg/day).

Single dose of 0.4 mg/kg or more may be given intermittently (biweekly or monthly).

Aim toward lower end of ranges with heavy marrow infiltration by tumor cells.

Indications:

Chronic lymphocytic leukemia, occasionally lymphoma including Hodgkin's disease (when long-term management needed).

Toxicities:

Bone Marrow—neutropenia, lymphopenia, and thrombocytopenia (lasting up to 10–14 days after treatment stopped) dosage

dependent, especially if cumulative dose reaches 6.5 mg/kg
during a continuous program—rarely effects are irreversible.

Gastrointestinal—nausea and vomiting, diarrhea, mucositis generally
only at high doses.

Miscellaneous—jaundice due to hepatic toxicity, fever, rash,
pulmonary fibrosis, peripheral neuropathy, cystitis, gonadal
hypofunction, seizures (all rare).

Precautions:

Observe blood counts at regular intervals (no more than 2 weeks
apart) in patients on continuous therapy, and adjust doses if
counts fall below normal.

Be wary of patients undergoing radiation therapy within 4 weeks of
chlorambucil treatment as they may have more profound marrow
sensitivity.

CIS-DIAMMINEDICHLOROPLATINUM
(C-DDP; Cisplatin®)

Physical Properties and Mechanisms:

Heavy metal compound which in aqueous solution becomes a
positively charged molecule.

Combines with sites on DNA, RNA, or protein to form covalent
links analagous to alkylating reactions.

May form intrastrand crosslinks in DNA.

Dosage:

50–150 mg/m^2 IV (often in divided doses), or 20 mg/m^2 IV q day × 5;
cycle repeated q 3–4 weeks.

Indications:

Testicular, ovarian, head and neck, breast, prostate, lung,
esophageal, and bladder carcinoma. Also employed with variable
results in many other tumors.

Toxicities:

Renal—dysfunction usually starts the second week after a dose—
other nephrotoxins (e.g. aminoglycosides) may contribute to
toxicity.

Electrolyte—lowering of serum Na^+, K^+, Ca^{++}, and especially
Mg^{++}.

Neurologic—peripheral neuropathy (including nerve deafness,
paresthesias, loss of proprioception and vibration, loss of taste)
more common with higher doses—also seizures, optic neuritis,
blurred vision.

Gastrointestinal—nausea/vomiting common in first 24 hours, occasionally up to a week later.

Bone Marrow—myelosuppression moderate (nadirs of WBC, platelets usually d. 14–21).

Allergic Reactions—1–2% (epinephrine, antihistamines, corticosteroids may be helpful).

Precautions:

Renal function should be adequate prior to administration of C-DDP.

Hydration necessary (keep urine output between 150–200 cc/hr. for at least 2–3 hrs. prior to administration and minimum of 6–8 hours after treatment).

Use caution with patients already experiencing impaired hearing, myelosuppression, or previous C-DDP sensitivity.

Comments:

C-DDP may be more effective in the presence of calcium channel blockers.

CYCLOPHOSPHAMIDE
(Cytoxan®)

Physical Properties and Mechanisms:

Synthetic agent chemically related to the nitrogen mustards.

Well absorbed orally.

Alkylator, with active metabolite in low doses preferentially toxic to lymphocytes.

Dosage:

500–750 mg/m² IV (usually at 3–4 week intervals) 1–5 mg/kg/day p.o.

Indications:

Lymphoma; breast, ovarian, lung, and prostate carcinomas.

Toxicities:

Bone Marrow—moderate suppression 7–14 days after treatment.

Bladder—hemorrhagic cystitis rare, and usually vigorous hydration will avert this problem.

Gastrointestinal—nausea/vomiting mild.

Dermatologic—alopecia.

Cardiopulmonary—rare pulmonary interstitial fibrosis; or cardiac necrosis with high doses (greater than 1000 mg/m²).

Miscellaneous—inappropriate water retention, sterility.

Precautions:

Hydration advised with IV treatment (greater than 150 cc/hr for at least 2 hrs. before and 8 hours after treatment).

Furosemide appropriate for fluid retention. In situation of renal failure, serum half-life prolonged causing increased myelosuppression.

CYTOSINE ARABINOSIDE
(Cytarabine; ARA-C; Cytosar-U®)

Physical Properties and Mechanisms:

Synthetic nucleoside, differing from normal nucleoside cytidine, due to replacement of the sugar residue, ribose, with arabinose.

Primarily kills cells in S phase, less so by blocking progression of cells from G_1 and S.

Inhibits DNA polymerase; and by direct incorporation into DNA, it causes slowdown of chain elongation.

Rapid metabolism favors infusion as treatment of choice.

Potent immunosupppressant.

Dosage: (quite variable)

Usually 100 mg/m² (most favored)—200 mg/m² IV infusion (over 8–24 hrs.) per day up to 10 days or 1–3 gm/m² q 12 hrs for 8–12 doses.

30–100 mg/m² intrathecally q. 4 days until CSF clears.

20 mg/m² SQ for 7–21 days for chronic low dose treatment (e.g. certain myeloproliferative disorders).

Indications:

Acute leukemias, CML (blast phase), certain lymphomas (high grade).

Toxicities:

Bone Marrow—generalized suppression-WBC usually nadirs at day 7–9; a secondary deeper nadir may occur. Day 15–24 platelets nadir between day 12–15; megaloblastic changes.

Pulmonary—edema, sometimes associated with respiratory distress syndrome.

Gastrointestinal—nausea and vomiting moderate but common, mucositis common, diarrhea, ulcerations (including pneumatosis cystoides intestinalis), bowel necrosis rare.

Hepatic—mild liver function abnormalities common, rarely severe (in this case may be veno-occlusive type).

Neurologic—somnolence, coma, personality changes, headache (all uncommon), cerebellar dysfunction with high doses.

Urinary—retention rare.

Dermatologic—rash, alopecia, cellulitis at injection site, corneal toxicity (reversible), conjunctivitis.

Allergic—fever, anaphylaxis rare.

Cardiovascular—cardiomyopathy in high dose situations when used with cyclophosphamide in marrow transplants; thrombophlebitis.

Precautions:

Blindness, paraplegia seen rarely with intrathecal administration.

Do not use diluent containing benzyl alcohol for intrathecal use.

"Cytarabine Syndrome"—fever, myalgias, occasionally chest pain, conjunctivitis occurring 6–12 hours after drug administration—steroids useful.

Monitor blood counts frequently after treatment and consider holding treatment if WBC ≤1000 and/or platelets ≤50,000.

Avoid overproduction of uric acid with rapid tumor lysis.

Pancreatitis may be seen in patients previously treated with asparaginase.

Comments:

Cytosine arabinoside may be safely administered intrathecally in close proximity to intrathecal methotrexate.

DTIC
(Dacarbazine; DTIC-Dome®)

Physical Properties and Mechanisms:

Hypotheses for action include:

1. Alkylation,
2. Inhibition of DNA synthesis by acting as purine analog,

or

3. Interaction with sulfhydryl groups.

Activated in liver; metabolic breakdown plus renal excretion.

Dosage:

150–300 mg/m^2 IV × 5 days every 3–4 weeks (may be lesser dosages used in certain combinations) or 375 mg/m^2 IV single dose.

Indications:

Melanoma, sarcomas, Hodgkin's disease.

Toxicities:

Bone Marrow Suppression—primarily leukopenia and thrombocytopenia, usually nadir between days 7–14.

Hepatic—hepatic vein thrombosis and necrosis rare but may be fatal.

Anaphylaxis—rare.

Gastrointestinal—greater than 90% patients with 1–12 hr. of nausea or vomiting following treatment.

Miscellaneous—flu-like syndrome with fever, myalgias lasting up to several days; rash and rare photosensitivity.

Precautions:

Extravasation may cause severe pain and tissue damage.

DOXORUBICIN
(Adriamycin®)

Physical Properties and Mechanisms:

Cytotoxic anthracycline antibiotic isolated from cultures of *Streptomyces*. Excreted 50% in bile. Binds to nucleic acids by intercalation of drug with double helix, inhibiting DNA synthesis.

Dosage:

50–75 mg/m² IV single dose every 3–4 weeks; 20 mg/m² IV weekly; 30 mg/m²/day × 3 days every 4 weeks.

Indications:

Leukemias, lymphomas, small cell lung carcinoma, sarcomas, neuroblastoma, Wilms' tumor; breast, ovarian, and bladder carcinomas.

Toxicities:

Cardiac—congestive heart failure, usually not ameliorated with conventional treatment—tachycardia may be early indicator—risk usually 1–2% if total dose less than 450 mg/m². Transient arrhythmias occasionally seen during or soon after treatment.

Bone Marrow—may be profound with leukocyte nadir usually at 10–14 days.

Gastrointestinal—frequent nausea and vomiting. Stomatitis infrequent, occur 5–10 days after treatment. Necrotizing colitis may occur in combinations with cytosine arabinoside.

Dermatologic—alopecia common.

Miscellaneous—radiation effects on tissues may be enhanced or recalled by Adriamycin.

Precautions:

Not recommended in patients with pre-existing congestive heart failure, or significant coronary artery disease.

Do not exceed 550 mg/m² total dose (or 400 mg/m² in those with prior mediastinal radiation or concurrent cyclophosphamide treatment—consider daunorubicin as additive to total dose).

Extravasation is usually locally damaging and should be treated according to appropriate extravasation protocols.

Urine may turn red for 1–2 days.

Check bilirubin prior to treatment and if elevated, reduce or hold dose.

5-FLUOROURACIL
(5-FU)

Physical Properties and Mechanisms:

Analogue of uracil with fluorine substitution at the 5 position.

Metabolized in liver and gastrointestinal mucosa.

Converted to nucleotide 5-FdUmP, which binds tightly to thymidylate synthetase, thus inhibiting DNA synthesis.

Also converted to fluorouridine triphosphate (FUTP), which inhibits RNA function.

Direct incorporation into DNA.

Methotrexate, when given prior to 5-FU, may increase 5-FU nucleotide formation.

Leucovorin given with 5-FU may stabilize the complex: 5-dUmp and thymidylate synthetase.

Dosage:

Intravenous schedules are variable. Some examples:

1. 500 mg/m² IV every week (bolus) or q day × 5 every 3 weeks.
2. 800–1200 IV mg/m² q day × 5 constant infusion.
3. 400 mg/m² IV q day × 10–30 days constant infusion.

May also be given intraarterially in similar dose range.

Indications:

Carcinomas of colon, breast, stomach, esophagus, pancreas and ovary.

Toxicities:

Bone Marrow—moderate—leukocyte nadir usually 9–14 days but may be as long as 20.

Mucositis—may appear after 5–7 days.

Gastrointestinal—nausea/vomiting uncommon—diarrhea transient.

Dermatologic—moderate alopecia, rash.

Miscellaneous—conjunctivitis; cerebellar ataxia rare and usually 3–4 weeks after beginning treatment.

Precautions:

Check blood counts and be sure WBC greater than 3500, platelets greater than 100,000 before next dose.

Dose modifications generally unnecessary with hepatic or renal dysfunction due to extrahepatic metabolism.

HYDROXYUREA
(Hydrea®)

Physical Properties and Mechanisms:
DNA synthesis inhibitor (mechanism uncertain); action
complementary with radiation therapy in experimental
situations—1) may be lethal for certain cells in S phase, 2) cells
exposed to hydroxyurea may stall in G_1 phase where they are
quite susceptible to radiation, 3) normal DNA repair process is
hindered by hydroxyurea.
Well absorbed orally; essentially cleared from circulation in 24 hours.

Dosage:
Continuous Treatment—20–30 mg/kg p.o. daily.
Intermittent Treatment—80 mg/kg p.o. every 3rd day. A six week
trial is generally considered sufficient to detect a response.

Indications:
Chronic myelogenous leukemia (CML), blast crisis of ANLL, ovarian
carcinoma, various tumors when combined with radiation therapy.

Toxicities:
Bone Marrow—leukopenia most profound, with rapid recovery once
drug stopped; less often thrombocytopenia, anemia;
megaloblastic changes.
Gastrointestinal—nausea, vomiting, diarrhea, constipation, stomatitis.
Dermatologic—rash, facial erythema.
Neurologic—headache, dizziness, hallucinations (all rare).
Hepatic—mild enzyme elevations.
Renal—mild azotemia (uncommon).

Precautions:
Hold treatment if WBC drops below 2500 or if platelet count 100,000.

IFOSFAMIDE
(Ifex®)

Physical Properties and Mechanisms:
Synthetic analogue of cyclophosphamide metabolically converted to
active intermediates that alkylate DNA.

Dosage:
1.2–1.6 gm/m^2 IV (over at least 30 min) q day 1–5 every 3–4 weeks
or up to 2400 mg/m^2/day as a 5-day continuous infusion or 3 gm/
m^2/d × 2 every 14–28 days.

Indications:
In combination with other agents for an expanding list of
malignancies, including testicular carcinoma, sarcomas.

Toxicities:

Hemorrhagic Cystitis—usually avoided by vigorous hydration, and a
  protector such as mesna ($\leq$6% incidence if used)
Bone Marrow—suppression moderate
CNS—(12% incidence) somnolence, confusion, hallucinations, usually
  reversible.
Miscellaneous—alopecia (83%), renal dysfunction (6%).

Precautions:

Marrow function should be adequate prior to administration (WBC
  $\geq$3000, platelets $\geq$75,000).
Assess urinalysis prior to each cycle—if >10 RBC per HPF, wait
  until this clears.
May interfere with wound healing.
Hydrate with at least 2 liters over each 24 hour period.

MESNA
(Mesnex™)

Physical Properties and Mechanisms:

Short-lived sulfhydryl compound which concentrates itself in the
  bladder and complexes with ifosfamide (or cyclophosphamide).
Specifically counteracts bladder toxin, acrolein, produced by
  breakdown of ifosfamide.

Dosage:

With constant infusion ifosfamide: Administer mesna (equal to 10% of
  the dose of ifosfamide) IV, 15 minutes prior to ifosfamide,
  followed by a 24 hour infusion equal to 100% of the ifosfamide
  dose (they are compatible in same solution).
With bolus or short infusion ifosfamide: Administer mesna at 20% of
  total dose of ifosfamide over 15–30 minutes starting 30 minutes
  prior to ifosfamide; repeat mesna at 4 and 8 hour points.

Toxicities:

Gastrointestinal—nausea/vomiting, diarrhea, altered taste sensation.
Miscellaneous—fatigue, headache, limb pain, hypotension, allergic
  reactions.

Precautions:

May give false positive result for urinary ketones.
Stable in solution with ifosfamide or cyclophosphamide but not with
  platinum.
If hematuria does not abate with mesna, would decrease or hold
  further ifosfamide.

MELPHALAN
(L-Phenylalanine Mustard; L-PAM; Alkeran®)

Physical Properties and Mechanisms:
Derivative of nitrogen mustard, acting as a bifunctional alkylator.

Dosage:
Usual dose 6 mg p.o. q. day for 2–3 weeks with readjustment after weekly blood counts. Maintenance daily dose approximately 2 mg. Alternatively, 0.15 mg/kg/day × 7, 0.2 mg/kg/day for 5, or 0.25 mg/kg/day for 4 days, every 4–6 weeks, adjusted for blood counts.

Indications:
Multiple myeloma, ovarian carcinoma.

Toxicities:
Bone Marrow—generally easily reversible suppression of all major elements.
Gastrointestinal—nausea, vomiting, oral ulcerations, and diarrhea, generally with high-dose regimens.
Miscellaneous—rash, allergic reaction, pulmonary fibrosis, vasculitis, alopecia, gonadal hypofunction.

Precautions:
Secondary leukemias are possible after chronic treatment.
Discontinue if WBC <3000 or platelets <100,000 until counts have recovered.
Azotemia is not a contraindication.
Patients undergoing other chemotherapy or radiation therapy within 4 weeks of starting melphalan may exhibit enhanced marrow suppression.

6-MERCAPTOPURINE
(Purinethol®)

Physical Properties and Mechanisms:
Purine analog with substitution of thiol group at 6' position.
Active state at nucleotide level by action of enzyme hypoxanthine-guanine phosphoribosyl transferase (HGPRT).
Ultimately inhibits de novo purine synthesis.
Erratic absorption by oral route.
Likely cross resistance with 6-thioguanine

Dosage:
80–100 mg/m² p.o. for 5 days or longer.

Indications:
Acute leukemias, chronic myelogenous leukemia.

Toxicities:
Bone Marrow—nadirs by 7 days and recover usually by 14 days after last dose. Affects all blood elements.
Gastrointestinal—mild reversible hepatotoxicity, mucositis, esophagitis, nausea, diarrhea, anorexia.
Immunologic—cell mediated immunity suppressed.

Precautions:
Allopurinol may inhibit metabolic breakdown of 6-mercaptupurine, thus causing increased toxicity (6-mercaptopurine dose should be lowered to 25% of usual level in this situation).
Monitor liver enzymes and bilirubin regularly while treatment continues.
Monitor blood counts at least weekly while on treatment.
Consider decreasing dose with renal failure.

METHOTREXATE

Physical Properties and Mechanisms:
Analog of folic acid (cellular uptake by existing normal active transport system for folates). Synthesis of purine nucleotides and thymidylate is dependent on a supply of one carbon groups carried by reduced tetrahydrofolates. An enzyme, dihydrofolate reductase, maintains the intracellular pool of folates in a reduced state—methotrexate inhibits dihydrofolate reductase, causing a pileup of oxidized forms, thus interfering with purine and thymidylate synthesis.
Once methotrexate is polyglutamated intracellularly, it may directly inhibit thymidylate synthetase and other enzymes.
Cytotoxic effects can be reduced by providing a reduced folate compound (e.g. calcium leucovorin) following administration of methotrexate.
Levels of 1×10^{-8}M inhibit pyrimidine synthesis and 1×10^{-7}M inhibits purine synthesis.

Dosage:
25–40 mg/m² IV, usually once or twice a month; up to 1500 mg/m² IV over 6–48 hrs. followed by leucovorin rescue, given at 3–4 weeks intervals; up to 25 mg/m² p.o. per dose.
Approximate dose 12 mg (total) intrathecally, given in normal saline over 1–5 minutes q 3–7 days for leukemic, lymphomatous, or carcinomatous meningitis. Since adequate

ventricular distribution by the lumbar route is unpredictable, an indwelling ventricular reservoir is advised as soon as feasible.

Indications:

Acute lymphocytic leukemia, non-Hodgkin's lymphoma, osteosarcoma, choriocarcinoma, breast carcinoma, head and neck and lung carcinomas.

Toxicities:

Bone Marrow—primarily WBC lowering, with nadirs from 5–14 days after treatment usually with rapid recovery.

Gastrointestinal—stomatitis also may occur from 5–14 days after treatment.

Renal—up to 10% have acute renal injuries on high-dose schedules, especially if they have not had attendant hydration and alkalinization of urine.

Hepatic—acute = usually within 1 week with increased enzymes, rapidly reversible. Chronic = with long-term oral treatment, up to 30% develop hepatic fibrosis, occasionally cirrhosis.

Pulmonary—acute, usually self-limited, with granulomas and eosinophilia on biopsy.

Neurologic—after intrathecal treatment (usually 3–4 doses) may see fever, cranial nerve palsies, motor dysfunction, coma, seizures (increased CSF protein, pressure, and pleiocytosis). Also acute arachnoiditis within 48 hrs. of injection.

In children—may see intracerebral calcifications, thinning of cortex, and ventricular dilatation when combined with radiation therapy.

Precautions:

Adequate renal function is vital since excretion is primarily via the kidney—if renal function inadequate, higher serum levels are maintained longer, thus increasing likelihood of toxicity. Consider advisability of use with other agents that may affect renal function (e.g. platinum).

Adequate wells of WBC, platelets advisable prior to treatment.

Methotrexate may accumulate and exit slowly from third space compartments such as ascites or effusions. Consider evaluating these collections prior to treatments.

Comments:

Methotrexate, while inhibiting purine synthesis, can augment 5-FU activation if given prior to 5-FU; 5-FU given before methotrexate, however, may block thymidylate synthetase and prevent the depletion of reduced folate pool by methotrexate. L-asparaginase may inhibit cytotoxic activity of methotrexate when given with or shortly after methotrexate.

MITOMYCIN
(Mutamycin®)
Physical Properties and Mechanisms:
  Antibiotic isolated from *Streptomyces*. Selective DNA inhibition by cross linking, and at high concentrations, may inhibit RNA and protein production. Cleared quickly by liver and peripheral metabolism.
Dosage:
  20 mg/m² IV every 6–8 weeks (as single agent).
Indications:
  In combination chemotherapy programs for gastric, pancreatic, and breast carcinomas.
Toxicities:
  Bone Marrow—leukopenia, thrombocytopenia may occur anytime up to 8 weeks after treatment (average 4 weeks)—produces cumulat ive myelosuppression and some do not recover fully.
  Skin and Mucous Membranes—4% with effects—cellulitis at injection site, stomatitis, rash, alopecia.
  Renal—2% with rise in creatinine.
  Pulmonary—diffuse interstitial infiltrates (rare).
  Gastrointestinal—moderate nausea/vomiting.
  Miscellaneous—Hemolytic-Uremic Syndrome: Sometimes fatal microangiopathic hemolytic anemia, thrombocytopenia, with renal failure and hypertension.
Precautions:
  Mitomycin is a vesicant and extravasation protocol required if it infiltrates.
  Aim for WBC ≥3500, platelets ≥100,000 prior to administration.

MITOXANTRONE
(Novantrone®)
Physical Properties and Mechanisms:
  Synthetic anthracenedione with structural resemblance to anthracyclines. May be a cycle non-specific intercalator with

DNA but probably more important is ability to cause DNA strand breaks.

Can condense DNA and RNA, and appear most effective in G_1 and G_2 phases. Slight renal and moderate biliary excretion.

Dosage:
12 mg/m^2 IV every day × 3 in acute leukemia. 10–14 mg/m^2 IV every 3–4 weeks in breast carcinoma.

Indications:
Acute non-lymphocytic leukemia, breast carcinoma.

Toxicities:
Bone Marrow—WBC usually nadir about 11 days after treatment; rarely severe unless prior chemotherapy or radiation therapy exposure.

Cardiac—congestive heart failure in 2–3% in doses up to 140 mg/m^2, especially if prior doxorubicin, mediastinal radiation, or cardiovascular disease.

Allergic—rare hypotension.

Dermatologic—phlebitis; extravasation can cause local injury; alopecia in 25%.

Gastrointestinal—nausea/vomiting in approximately 50%/stomatitis in 8% during first week—also diarrhea, dry mouth, abdominal pain.

Precautions:
May impart a blue-green color to urine and sclerae.

May precipitate if mixed with heparin/produces tissue irritation with extravasation.

NITROGEN MUSTARD
(Mechlorethamine; Mustargen®)

Physical Properties and Mechanisms:
Nitrogen analog of sulfur mustard/alkylating agent.

Dosage:
0.4 mg/kg IV as single or divided doses generally every 4 weeks.

Indications:
Hodgkin's disease, non-Hodgkin's lymphoma, chronic myelogenous and chronic lymphocytic leukemias.

Toxicities:
Bone Marrow—thrombocytopenia and granulocytopenia occur 6–8 days after treatment and may last 1½–3 weeks.

Gastrointestinal—moderate to severe nausea and vomiting (1–3 hrs. after administration) may last up to 24 hrs.

Miscellaneous—thrombosis or phlebitis in injected vein (avoid high concentration); rash, menstrual irregularity, sterility, jaundice, alopecia, vertigo, and tinnitus.

Precautions:

If local tissue infiltration (including external skin, eye, or inhalation exposure) potentially damaging tissue injury may follow (consult extravastion procedure).

May cause profound marrow suppression when coupled with radiation therapy.

Adequate bone marrow function required prior to administration.

PROCARBAZINE
(Matulane®)

Physical Properties and Mechanisms:

Hydrazine derivative proposed as an inhibitor of DNA, RNA, and protein synthesis.

Metabolized in liver and kidneys.

Crosses blood-brain barrier.

Dosage:

100 mg/m^2 p.o. × 14 days (often given every 4 weeks)

Indications:

Generally in advanced Hodgkin's disease as part of MOPP regimen (nitrogen mustard, vincristine, procarbazine, prednisone).

Toxicities:

Bone Marrow—general suppression 2–8 weeks after start of treatment, also rarely eosinophilia, hemolytic anemia.

Gastrointestinal—nausea and vomiting, occasionally jaundice, stomatitis, dry mouth, melena, diarrhea or constipation, abdominal pain.

Cardiovascular—hypotension, tachycardia.

Pulmonary—pneumonitis, effusions.

Neurologic—convulsions, ataxia, neuropathy, headache, confusion.

Ophthalmic—diplopia, papilledema, photophobia.

Urologic—hematuria, frequency.

Miscellaneous—allergic reactions, hallucinations, nightmares, myalgias.

Precautions:

Monitor blood counts, hepatic and renal function at regular intervals.

Antihistamines, antihypertensive agents, narcotics, phenothiazines, or barbiturates may potentiate CNS effects.

Ethanol ingestion may result in Antabuse-like phenomenon.

Procarbazine has monoamine oxidase activity, and tricyclic antidepressants, sympathomimetic agents, foods rich in tyramine (wine, yogurt, ripe cheese, bananas) should be avoided.

Gonadal hypofunction and secondary malignancies possible.

Advise patients to inform health-care providers of all medications used.

6-THIOGUANINE
(Thioguanine)

Physical Properties and Mechanisms:

Analog of guanine with substitution of thiol group at 6' position.

Active state at nucleotide level by action of enzyme hypoxanthine-guanine phosphoribosyl transferase (HGPRT).

Ultimately inhibits de novo purine synthesis.

Causes DNA strand breaks and greater sensitivity to alkylation.

Erratic absorption by oral route.

Likely cross-resistance with 6-mercaptopurine.

Dosage:

2–3 mg/kg/day p.o. for 5 days or longer.

Indications:

Acute non-lymphocytic leukemias.

Toxicities:

Bone Marrow—nadirs by 7 days and recovery usually by 14 days after last dose.

Gastrointestinal—rarely mild reversible hepatotoxicity (cholestatic type)—mild mucositis, esophagitis, nausea, anorexia.

Immunologic—cell mediated immunity suppressed.

Precautions:

Monitor blood counts at least weekly during treatment.

Monitor liver function tests regularly.

VINBLASTINE
(Velban®)

Physical Properties and Mechanisms:

Salt of an alkaloid from periwinkle herb/interferes with metabolic amino acid pathways/may interfere with mitotic spindle apparatus.

Dosage:

3.7–7.5 mg/m^2 IV at 1–4 week intervals.

Indications:

Hodgkin's and non-Hodgkin's lymphomas; testicular and breast carcinomas, choriocarcinoma, Kaposi's sarcoma.

Toxicities:

Bone Marrow—WBC nadir 5–10 days after dose and recover in 7–14 days—thrombocytopenia less common and with quicker recovery.

Pulmonary—bronchospasms seen, especially when vinblastine combined with mitomycin.

Gastrointestinal—abdominal pain and ileus (mimicking an acute abdominal event) most dramatic—nausea/vomiting uncommon—also constipation and pharyngitis.

Neurologic—peripheral neuropathy with paresthesias, loss of deep tendon reflexes; also headache, convulsions, mental depression.

Miscellaneous—malaise, skin vesiculations, dizziness.

Precautions:

Vesicant damage to local tissues with infiltration (consult extravasation procedure), including the eye if splashed.

Comments:

If used with bleomycin, it is suggested the vinblastine be given 6–8 hrs. before bleomycin, since the latter is active in metaphase.

VINCRISTINE
(Oncovin®)

Physical Properties and Mechanisms:

Salt of an alkaloid from the periwinkle herb—may cause metaphase arrest in mitosis.

Dosage:

1.4 mg/m^2 IV (maximum dose is 2 mg!) in adults at 1 week or longer intervals.

Indications:

Acute leukemias, non-Hodgkin's lymphomas, Hodgkin's disease, rhabdomyosarcoma, neuroblastoma, Wilms' tumor.

Toxicities:

Bone Marrow—very mild effect.

Neuropathy—peripheral neuropathy with sensory loss, paresthesias, especially decrease in deep tendon reflexes, difficulty walking— usually improves by 6th week following treatment—extraocular and laryngeal muscles may be affected.

Pulmonary—bronchospasm, especially when combined with mitomycin.

Gastrointestinal—abdominal pain associated with ileus and constipation.

Miscellaneous—moderate hair loss, convulsions (rare), inappropriate ADH syndrome, myalgias, dysuria, urinary retention.

Precautions:

Patients with demyelinating diseases, especially Charcot-Marie-Tooth syndrome, should not receive vincristine.

Vincristine should never be given intrathecally.

Allopurinol should be given prior to chemotherapy in leukemias and lymphomas to avoid serious uric acid buildup.

Avoid extravasation or eye exposure, since the agent can be locally damaging (consult extravasation procedure).

Routine bowel stimulants or stool softeners suggested for 1–2 weeks after each treatment or on a regular basis.

VP-16
(Etoposide, Epipodophyllotoxin, Vepesid®)

Physical Properties and Mechanism:

Semisynthetic derivative of podophyllotoxin inhibits nucleoside transport during G2 and S phases in particular, plus causing metaphase arrest.

Synergistic with C-DDP in experimental tumor systems.

Oral dose is twice the usual IV dose/cleared by renal, biliary, and metabolic processes.

Dosage:

35–100 mg/m^2 IV daily for 3–5 days (given slowly over 60–120 minutes to avoid hypotension) at 3–4 week intervals. Capsules (50 mg) given at twice the IV dose.

Indications:

Testicular, ovarian, and lung carcinomas; lymphomas.

Toxicities:

Bone Marrow—granulocyte nadirs 7–14 days after treatment; platelets nadir 9–16 days recovery usually complete by day 20 (non-cumulative suppression).

Allergic—0.7–2.0% with chills, fever, bronchospasm, or hypotension.

Neurologic—mild neurotoxicity rare.

Gastrointestinal—mild to moderate nausea/vomiting in 1/3 (slightly more frequent with oral administration).

Dermatologic—alopecia in 2/3 (generally reversible).

Precautions:

Agent should not come in contact with skin (wash immediately).

Intravenous solutions should contain 0.2–0.4 mg/ml (above 0.4 may result in precipitation).

Hormonal Agents

FLUTAMIDE
(Eulexin®)

Physical Properties and Mechanisms:
Non-steroidal antiandrogen. Inhibits androgen uptake and/or nuclear
  binding in target tissues. May elevate plasma testosterone and
  estradiol levels.

Dosage:
250 mg (two capsules) orally 3 × a day.

Indications:
In combination with LHRH analogues (such as leuprolide acetate) in the
  treatment of metastatic prostate carcinoma.

Toxicities: (in association with LHRH agonist)
Bone Marrow—rare myelosuppresion
Renal—rare increase in creatinine.
Gastrointestinal—diarrhea (12%), nausea/vomiting (11%), anorexia (4%)
Miscellaneous—hot flashes (61%), loss of libido (36%), impotence (33%),
  gynecomastia (9%), hypertension (1%), CNS effects (1%).

Precautions:
May reduce sperm counts.

LEUPROLIDE
(Lupron®)

Physical Properties and Mechanisms:
Potent synthetic analog of gonadotropin releasing hormone (LHRH).
Inhibitor of gonadotropin secretion (and resultant ovarian and testicular
  steroid synthesis) when given continuously.
Brief initial stimulation of LHRH reverses and at 2–4 weeks, inhibitory
  effect is complete.

Dosage:
Aqueous solution 1 mg (0.2 cc) subcutaneously daily; suspension (acetate
  salt) 7.5 mg IM monthly.

Indications:
Prostate (in place of orchiectomy) and breast carcinomas.

Toxicities:
Cardiovascular—edema
Central Nervous System—dizziness, pain, headache, paresthesia.
Endocrine—breast tenderness or enlargement, hot flashes, impotence.

Gastrointestinal—anorexia, constipation, nausea and vomiting, diarrhea.

Dermatologic—erythema at injection site, rash, hair loss.

Miscellaneous—fatigue, fever, facial swelling, myalgias, sour taste, decreased memory.

Precautions:

Watch for flare of disease at start of treatment, especially if cord compression possible.

Vehicle for leuprolide is benzyl alcohol, to which some are allergic.

MEGESTROL ACETATE
(Megace®)

Physical Properties and Mechanisms:

Antiluteinizing effect mediated by pituitary is postulated in endometrial carcinoma, but effect in breast carcinoma uncertain.

Dosage:

Usual 40–320 mg orally per day in divided doses, but up to 800 mg per day have safely been given.

Indications:

Palliative treatment of advanced breast carcinoma or endometrial carcinoma. Also used as an appetite stimulant.

Toxicities:

Relatively common: weight gain, edema. Rare: alopecia, carpal tunnel syndrome, thrombophlebitis.

Precautions:

Long-term administration in dogs (up to 7 yrs.) resulted in increased benign and malignant mammary tumors. Not recommended during pregnancy.

TAMOXIFEN
(Nolvadex®)

Physical Properties and Mechanisms:

Nonsteroidal "antiestrogen"

May exhibit effect by binding to estrogen receptors.

Presence of estrogen receptors in adequate amounts is likely to be predictive of tumor response.

Dosage:

10 mg. orally twice a day.

Indications:

Breast carcinoma; occasionally prostate carcinoma.

Toxicities:

Flare reaction—increase in bone pain (hypercalcemia may also occur) and malaise, often associated with early tumor response— corticosteroid helpful symptomatically.

Bone Marrow—rare leukopenia, thrombocytopenia.

Ocular—rare retinopathy and decrease in visual acuity.

Neurologic—rare dizziness, headache.

Miscellaneous—relatively common: hot flashes. Uncommon: nausea/vomiting, vaginal bleeding or discharge, edema, distaste for food, pruritus vulvae, depression. Also, potential increase in thromboembolic events.

Precautions:

Use not advised in pregnancy.

Chapter 11

Biologic Response Modifiers

In recent years considerable efforts have been made to develop systemic treatment strategies other than cytotoxic chemotherapy. A particularly exciting and innovative area encompasses efforts to manipulate the human immune system, in order to deter the progression of malignancy. Despite the vast and bewildering complexity of the immune network, significant developments have enabled clinicians to induce true responses in human tumors. Utilizing new technologies (such as recombinant DNA methodology), researchers have been able to produce large quantities of biologic substances, which are ordinarily present only in minute amounts during normal physiologic situations.

Current understanding of the interrelationships in the immune system has focused on two general topics: cellular elements and cytokines (hormonal secretions causing multiple effects on cells inside and outside the immune network). Although cells and their products function in a coordinated manner, it is helpful to consider them separately.

Macrophages are considered to be initiators in many of the cellular responses to antigenic material, as these cells process antigen in order to present it to lymphocytes (macrophages also appear to have non-specific antineoplastic properties, which are poorly understood). Thymus-derived (T) lymphocytes then mount a specific reaction to the antigen as long as they recognize certain major histocompatibility (MHC) molecules in association with the antigen; two major classes of T lymphocytes are known to react with different MHC molecules. Those T lymphocytes bearing the CD8 marker recognize class I MHC (HLA-A, HLA-B, HLA-C) determinants, while CD4 bearing T lymphocytes recognize Class II MHC determinants (HLA-D). Since a large number of possible combinations exist, the heterogeneity and complexity of the immune response resides here.

Following the initial cellular interaction with antigen, other events follow. A host of cells including other macrophages, T lymphocytes, B (bursal equivalent) lymphocytes, and other lymphocyte types are recruited to proliferate and differentiate, thus fulfilling a reaction (and subsequent recognition) related to the given antigen. Finally, a suppressor network is engaged to allow modulation of the reaction.

Certain specialized lymphocytes have specific activities. Natural killer (NK) cells are lymphocytes capable of destroying certain human tumor cells without the advantage of prior exposure. Lymphokine activated (or LAK) cells can acquire the ability to kill a variety of fresh human tumor cells if exposed to a specific lymphokine, interleukin-2 (IL-2) Similarly, lymphocytes invading malignant tumors (tumor infiltrating lymphocytes, or TIL cells) have been isolated, exposed to IL-2, and have been found to be even more potent effector cells than LAK cells.[1]

Cytokines constitute the second major area for potential clinical benefits in tumor immunotherapy. Some substances are directly toxic to tumor cells (e.g. tumor necrosis factor or TNF, and lymphotoxin), while others primarily influence specific cellular activities (e.g. IL-2) or may combine direct cytotoxic effects on tumor cells with immune cell stimulation (e.g. the interferons). Some current treatment strategies involving the immune system will be summarized next.

THE INTERFERONS

Discovered in 1957 as an antiviral substance of uncertain nature, interferons are now known to be a family of glycoproteins, synthesized by a wide variety of cells in the human. The alpha (α) and beta (β) varieties are potential products of most human cells but gamma (γ) interferon is made only by certain T cells and large granular lymphocytes. Stimuli for interferon production include viral infection, chemical inducers, and immune stimulation in general. Effects are mediated via specific receptors: alpha and beta interferons share a common receptor, while gamma has a unique counterpart.

The interferons are believed to have myriad and diverse actions on transformed cells. They may induce and modulate expression of Class I (and II) major histocompatibility antigens, thus facilitating recognition by cytotoxic T lymphocytes; in similar fashion, the expression of other membrane structures, including tumor associated antigens, may be increased due to interferon's effects on the tumor cell cytoskeleton.[2] Another mechanism of action is inhibition of oncogenes and growth factors like platelet derived growth factors (PDGF) and epidermal growth factor (EGF).[3,4] As a result of PDGF inhibition, expression of the c-myc and c-fos oncogenes may be attenuated.[5] Interferons may also induce differentiation (or reversal of transformation) of cells in vitro.[6]

Interferons also directly affect the functional activities of various immune effector cells. Macrophages develop an increase in F_c receptors and phagocytic capacities after exposure, especially to gamma interferon.[7]

Natural killer and LAK cells are also stimulated by interferons, which may augment the activities of other lymphokines such as IL-2.[8] Interferons may convert Pre-NK cells to fully functional counterparts while accelerating their kinetics and recycling.[9,10] B cells have variable behavior after interferon exposure, apparently depending on dose and exposure time.[11]

In the treatment of human malignancy the most dramatic examples of interferon's success have been in hairy cell leukemia (HCL) and chronic myelogenous leukemia (CML). Low doses of alpha interferon are usually effective in up to 95% of HCL patients, resulting in fewer infectious complications and improved survival. The response to treatment may be delayed 4–6 months, and the granulocyte count is usually the first to improve. Patients with CML will often have improvement in their peripheral blood picture, but true complete remissions are rare. Other malignancies that may respond favorably to treatment with interferons include nodular (indolent) lymphomas, T cell lymphomas, multiple myeloma, AIDS-related Kaposi's sarcoma, renal cell carcinoma, melanoma, ovarian carcinoma, and gliomas.[12]

Interferon treatment is not devoid of side-effects, and flu-like symptoms (fatigue, fever, anorexia, rigors) are moderate to severe in about 50% of patients; they are reversible with discontinuation of interferon. Other symptoms noted in lesser frequencies include somnolence and confusion (more common in elderly), nausea and vomiting (up to 50%), diarrhea (25%), asymptomatic hypotension and tachycardia, myalgias, abdominal pain, rash, and pruritus. Transient leukopenia and elevated transaminases may also be noted.

The recommended dose of alpha-interferon for HCL is 2 million units/m²
IM or subcutaneously three days a week. In other tumors dosages up to
15 million units/m² have been used, and both the frequency of side effects
and the efficacy tend to increase at higher dose ranges.

Future efforts with interferons will include coordinating its use with
other cytokines, with chemotherapy, and with radiation therapy.

INTERLEUKIN-2 (IL-2) AND LAK CELLS

With the advent of gene cloning techniques, the gene for IL-2 has been
isolated and expressed in Escherichia coli, allowing the clinical use of this
versatile substance. Interleukin-2 has multiple effects on the immune network, including stimulating growth and differentiation of activated T
cells, inducing heightened cytotoxicity in NK cells, and stimulating B cell
development.[13]

Lymphoid cells obtained by leukopheresis and incubated in vitro with
IL-2 emerge as cells (LAK cells) capable of killing fresh tumor cells, and
these cells can be reinfused back into patients to mediate anti-tumor effects (adoptive immunotherapy). A typical treatment schedule might start
with intermittent boluses of IL-2 (10,000–100,000 units/kg body weight)
given IV to a patient every 8 hours for 5 days (infusions have also been
used). Two days later leukopheresis is done daily for 5 days, with a typical
yield of $5 \times 10^9 - 3 \times 10^{10}$ lymphocytes per day. These cells are then incubated with IL-2 for 5 days, and subsequently reinfused with more IL-2
into the patient. A treatment cycle takes about 3 weeks.[14]

Of the first 55 patients treated at the National Cancer Institute 21
responded, 5 being complete responses.[14] Since then the treatment has
been applied to specific tumors, most notably renal cell carcinoma and
melanoma (up to 10% complete responses and 20% partial responses).
Continuing efforts to maximize therapeutic effects include selection of
patients in high risk adjuvant settings where initial tumor bulk is not so
high.

One major drawback is the considerable toxicity associated with treatment. A profound capillary leak syndrome leading to multiple organ dysfunction and fluid retention can be life threatening. Hypotension, azotemia, and pulmonary infiltrates are associated with this syndrome, and
mortality related to treatment is about 2%.

LEVAMISOLE

Levamisole is a synthetic phenylimidazothiazole which has properties of a non-specific immune stimulant. Recent clinical results have indicated a beneficial role for the combination of levamisole and 5-fluorouracil in the adjuvant treatment of Dukes C colon carcinoma.[15] The dose of levamisole was 150 mg orally for 3 consecutive days every two weeks for a year. Side effects include nausea, vomiting, diarrhea, infrequent myelosuppression, and dermatitis.

MONOCLONAL ANTIBODIES

A relatively new technology with vast potential is the production of monoclonal antibodies (MoAbs). Pioneered by Kohler and Milstein,[16] countless single antibody sources have been developed, usually from mice immunized with specific tumor extracts (the details of the process are beyond the scope of this chapter, but reviews are readily available).[17]

Monoclonal antibodies, due to their relative specificity for tumor tissue, can be labeled with tracer substances and used for detecting small tumor deposits.[18] Alternatively, they can be used therapeutically to localize tumors and enhance immune destruction of malignant cells,[19] or with the aid of associated radiotherapeutic (e.g. [131]I) or chemical (e.g. ricin) moieties bound to them, monoclonal antibodies may directly mediate cellular destruction. In addition, these antibodies can complex with and perturb certain receptor functions (e.g. epidermal growth factor receptors[20]), thus interrupting growth stimulatory pathways available to malignant cells. Efforts to locate more efficient antibody forms have led to the formation of heteroantibodies and chimeric antibodies; ideally these antibodies will have optimal specificity for the tumor cells on one end and superior recognition capacity for an effector cell on the other.[21] While still in the formative stages, this technology has already shown promising results in various malignancies.[22,23]

REFERENCES

1. Rosenberg, S.A., Packard, B.S., Aebersold, P.M., et al: Use of tumor infiltrating lymphocytes and interleukin-2 in the immunotherapy of patients with metastatic melanoma. A preliminary report. *N Engl J Med* 319:1676, 1988.

2. Goldstein, D., Laszlo J.: Interferon therapy in cancer: from imaginon to interferon. *Cancer Res* 46:4315, 1986.

3. Revel M.: The interferon system in man: nature of the interferon molecules and mode of action In Becker, Y. (ed): *Antiviral Drugs and Interferon*. New York, Martinus Nijhoff, 1984, p. 358.

4. Taylor-Papadimitriou, J.: Effects of interferon on cell growth and function. *Interferon* 2:13, 1980.

5. Kimchi, A., Einat, M. Resnitzky, D.: Antagonistic effect of interferon and platelet derived growth factor on gene expression. In Dianzani F., Rossi, G.B. (eds): *The Interferon System*. New York, Raven Press, 1985, p. 429.

6. Hicks, N.J., Morris, A.G., Burke, D.C.: Partial reversion of the transformed phenotype of murine sarcoma virus-transformed cells in the presence of interferon: A possible mechanism for the antitumor effect of interferon. *J Cell Sci* 49:225, 1981.

7. Guyre, P.M., Morganelli, P.M., Miller, R.: Recombinant immune interferon increases immunoglobulin G F_c receptors on cultured human mononuclear phagocytes. *J Clin Invest* 72:393, 1983.

8. Vilcek, J., Kelke, H.C., Jumming, L.E., Yip Y.K.: Structure and function of human interferon gamma. In Ford, R.J. (ed): *Mediators in Cell Growth and Differentiation*. New York, Raven Press, 1985, p. 299.

9. Bloom, B.R.: Interferon and the immune system. *Nature* 284:593, 1980.

10. Saksela E., Timonen, T., Cantell, K.: Human natural killer cell activity is augmented by interferon via recruitment of "pre NK cells." *Scand J Immunol* 10:257, 1979.

11. Braun, W., Levy, H.B.: Interferon preparations as modifiers of immune responses. *Proc Soc Exp Biol Med* 141:769, 1972.

12. Clark, J.W., Longo, D.L.: Interferons in cancer therapy. In DeVita, V.T. Jr., Hellman, S., Rosenberg, S.A. (eds): *Cancer: Principles and Practice of Oncology Updates*, 2nd ed. Philadelphia, J.B. Lippincott, 1987, p. 1.

13. Smith, K.A.: Interleukin-2: inception, impact, and implication. *Science* 240:1169, 1988.

14. Rosenberg, S.A., Lotze, M.T., Muul, L.M., et al: Observations on the systematic administration of autologous lymphokine activated killer cells and recombinant interleukin-2 to patients with metastatic cancer. *N Engl J Med* 313:1485, 1985.

15. Laurie, J.A., Moertel, C.G., Fleming, T.R., et al: Surgical adjuvant therapy of large bowel carcinoma: An evaluation of levamisole and the combination of levamisole and 5-fluorouracil. A study of the North Central Cancer Treatment Group and Mayo Clinic. *J Clin Oncol* 1447–1456, 1989.

16. Kohler, G., Milstein, C.: Continuous cultures of fused cells secreting antibodies of predefined specificity. *Nature* 256:495, 1975.

17. Dillman, R.O.: Monoclonal antibodies for treating cancer. *Ann Intern Med* 111:592, 1989.

18. Engelstad, B.L., Spitler, L.E., Del Rio, M.J., et al: Phase I immunolym-phoscintigraphy with an In-111-labeled antimelanoma monoclonal antibody. *Radiology* 161:419, 1986.
19. Brown, S.L., Miller, R.A., Horning, S.J.: Treatment of B-cell lymphomas with anti-idiotype antibodies alone and in combination with alpha-interferon. *Blood* 73:651, 1989.
20. Rodeck, U., Herlyn, M., Herlyn, D., et al: Tumor growth modulation by a monoclonal antibody to the epidermal growth factor receptor: immunologically mediated and effector cell-independent effects. *Cancer Res* 47:3692, 1987.
21. Reichmann, L., Clark, M.R., Waldmann, H., et al: Reshaping antibodies for therapy. *Nature* 332:323, 1988.
22. Press, O.W., Eary, J.F., Badger, C.C., et al: Treatment of refractory non-Hodgkin's lymphoma with radiolabeled MB-1 (Anti-CD37) antibody. *J Clin Oncol* 7:1027, 1989.
23. Hale, G., Dyeer, M.J., Waldmann, H., et al: Remission induction in non-Hodg-kin's lymphoma with reshaped human monoclonal antibody CAMPATH-1H. *Lancet* 2:1384, 1988.

Chapter 12

Complications of Cancer and Cancer Treatment

FEVER IN THE CANCER PATIENT

One of the most common and dangerous clinical dilemmas in caring for cancer patients relates to the issues of fever and infection. There are numerous reasons why cancer patients are more vulnerable to infection, including the breakdown of normal tissue barriers, hypogammaglobulinemia, defective cell mediated immunity, post-splenectomy states, and qualitative derangements in leukocyte function due to exposure to corticosteroids, chemotherapy, and other drugs; perhaps the most powerful determinant, however, is granulocytopenia related to treatments with chemotherapy or radiation.

Fever may result from inflammation of various organs, drug reactions, transfusions, and tumor breakdown, but in the majority of cases, it is related to a true infection. A significant fever may be defined as one temperature elevation above 38.5°C (101.3°F) or two to three elevations above 38°C (100.4°F) in a 24 hour period. Not all episodes of infection will declare themselves as plainly, especially if medications (e.g. corticosteroids, anti-inflammatory agents) mask the febrile reaction. In a setting of neutropenia (defined as <500 PMN's or bands per microliter) or with a rapidly falling WBC level, fever is an ominous sign, and the promptness of treatment may determine the outcome. A high index of suspicion is necessary in patients with unexplained new lethargy or hypotension since neutropenic patients may not exhibit the usual signs of inflammation. Approximately 30–35% of granulocytopenic patients will develop an infection, as the duration of granulocytopenia and the integrity of their phagocytic reserves play key roles.[1]

The first step in addressing a fever or suspected infection is to assess the patient's history and physical examination for clues to determine the source:

1. In general, search for specific localizing new symptoms or signs.
2. Special attention should be given to the following:

    a. Respiratory tract symptoms and findings;
    b. Optic fundi;
    c. Sinus, mouth, and teeth: tenderness, drainage or inflammation;
    d. Perianal tenderness; and
    e. New skin lesions or inflammation, especially at sites of catheter insertion.

The next step is to assess specific symptomatic areas with appropriate tests and cultures. General workup would include:

1. Biopsy or aspiration of suspicious skin lesions, catheter (and Omaya reservoir) exit sites;
2. Minimum of 2 sets of blood cultures from peripheral vein and indwelling venous access catheters;
3. Chest x-ray; and
4. Urinalysis and culture.

Most infections (80% or more) arise from endogenous flora, although an individual's endogenous flora may become quite different when he or she is hospitalized, at which time Gram-negative organisms commonly replace Gram-positive counterparts. Risk factors for oropharyngeal colonization include alcoholism, diabetes, coma, malnutrition, azotemia, and the use of endotracheal or nasogastric tubes.[2] In addition, antacids and H_2 blockers may increase gastric pH enough to allow greater growth of Gram-negative organisms, thus heightening the chance of tracheal colonization (sucralfate fortunately will not do this)[2]. Initial infections are fairly closely divided between Gram-negative and Gram-positive bacteria, as the incidence of *Pseudomonas* infection is mysteriously declining and *Staphylococcal* infection rates seem to be increasing (particularly with the use of venous access catheters). Common Gram-positive isolates include staphylococci (*S. epidermidis* is common in catheter-related infections), and streptococci (*Streptococcus. bovis* is associated with colon carcinoma) while Gram-negative representatives include *Escherichia. Coli*, *Pseudomonas*, and *Klebsiella* frequently. Fungal infections usually involve *Candida*, *Aspergillus*, *Cryptococcus*, or the Phycomycetes (*Mucor* and *Rhizopus*). Viral illnesses are often related to *herpes simplex, herpes zoster*, or *cytomegalovirus* (especially in bone marrow transplant recipients), among others.

Unless another source for fever is virtually certain (e.g. transfusion reaction), antibiotic treatment should start immediately. Once the decision has been made to institute broad spectrum antibiotics, consider the following steps:

1. Within 2 hours of a written order (or 20 minutes if patient is hypotensive or has meningitis), make sure antibiotics are administered.
2. Write orders legibly, and label them STAT. Note beeper number on orders.
3. Communicate verbally with the appropriate nurse and unit secretary.

Broad spectrum coverage with high bactericidal activity is very important in order to cover as many pathogens as is reasonable; generally one should aim for an *effective combination* that is the least toxic, the least expensive, and as restricted as possible in its spectrum of activity. Knowing the profile of pathogens present in a particular institution (get this information) is crucial in designing the most effective and economical therapy. House officers should be familiar with this type of profile for their own institution.

There are numerous effective broad spectrum regimens, yet most centers are employing either two- or three-drug combinations, containing an aminoglycoside (gentamicin, tobramycin, amikacin) and a cephalosporin or an antipseudomonas penicillin (mezlocillin, piperacillin, azlocillin) or both. Although some broad spectrum single agents may well be as effective as the combinations, the ability of various bacteria (especially. Gram-negative organisms) to develop resistant strains when treated with single agents argues for multiple antibiotic coverage in the compromised host.

Aminoglycosides form a group of agents with wide coverage of Gram-negative organisms but lesser activity against Gram-positive species, especially enterococci and streptococci. Aminoglycosides share a propensity for nephrotoxicity and ototoxicity and should be monitored for peak and trough levels (e.g. tobramycin should be maintained at serum levels between 4 and 12 mcg/ml). Amikacin is usually reserved for Gram-negative infections resistant to gentamicin and tobramycin.

The cephalosporins constitute a large family of medications with broad activity against both Gram-positive and Gram-negative species. There are some distinct differences in this group of agents: cephalothin possesses the best Gram-positive activity of the cephalosporins; ceftazidime (a third generation cephalosporin) has the highest activity against *Pseudomonas*. It is considered risky to substitute a cephalosporin for a penicillin if there is a history of urticaria, pruritus, or bronchospasm with penicillin; otherwise, ceftazadime is a reasonable choice.

The penicillins also form a diverse group. The semi-synthetic penicillins (nafcillin, oxacillin, methicillin) were developed to overcome the action of penicillinase-producing *Staphylococcus aureus* (if a non-penicillinase-producing staphylococcus is present, penicillin G is the choice; if a resistant strain, vancomycin would be used). Ticarcillin and carbenicillin possess good activity against anaerobes, *Pseudomonas*, and other Gram-negative bacteria; combined with an aminoglycoside, they may act synergistically (they should not, however, be infused together, as the aminoglycoside could be inactivated in solution). Extended spectrum penicillins (azlocillin, mezlocillin, piperacillin) are even more active against aerobic Gram-negative bacteria compared to carbenicillin and ticarcillin. They also have the advantages of better coverage with *Klebsiella* and enterococcus, less sodium loading, and less bleeding time prolongation, but are still not effective against penicillinase-producing staphylococci.[3] Piperacillin is often reserved to treat *Pseudomonas* resistant to mezlocillin and ceftazadime.

Special situations occur where other strategies are quite successful. Depending on the clinical situation, one may use a single agent for initial treatment, as ceftazadime, aztreonam (particularly in documented infections with aerobic Gram-negative rods not sensitive to aminoglycosides or mezlocillin) and imipenem (especially in documented serious mixed infections with anaerobes/aerobes) have been employed successfully in this manner. For suspected intra-abdominal sepsis an aminoglycoside and clindamycin provides excellent coverage. Suspected anaerobic infections (e.g. oral or perirectal sites) can be managed with clindamycin or metronidazole along with a broad spectrum agent.

The respiratory tract has been incriminated as the source in approximately 25% of febrile neutropenic episodes. If a localized patchy infiltrate is found with less than 14 days of neutropenia, it will most likely be bacterial in origin, while beyond 14 days fungal or viral etiologies increase in number. Provided the patient has an adequate platelet count (>50,000) a needle biopsy or bronchoscopy can provide an answer in about 1/2 the cases. Aspiration is one frequent cause of hospital acquired pneumonia, and ill patients with decreased gag and cough mechanisms may be predisposed further due to hypnotics, narcotics and neuroleptics—the possibility of bacterial colonization with virulent pathogens further compounds the problem. Clindamycin and penicillin are the leading choices for obvious aspiration, but a broader spectrum may be needed if the patient has been hospitalized for more than a few days.

Among other causal agents, *Legionella* and fungi can also cause patchy infiltrates. *Legionella* infection is often heralded by malaise with headache, followed by a non-productive cough several days later; diarrhea occurs in about 50% and neurologic changes or bradycardia are also frequent.[4] A rapid diagnosis can be made by direct fluorescent antibody on secretions, and by culture. Erythromycin and doxycycline are effective therapeutic agents. Fungal pneumonias are usually caused by *Candida* or *Aspergillus*. Checking the optic fundi may reveal the cottony white lesions associated with invasive candidiasis, but in general, histopathologic confirmation (open lung biopsy) is necessary to make a definitive diagnosis. *Aspergillus* can be diagnosed by bronchoalveolar lavage or by sputum analysis, and occasionally, a wedge shaped defect will be seen on chest x-ray suggestive of an infarction which may occur in *Aspergillus* pneumonia[5]. Amphotericin B is the drug of choice in these situations, and a cumulative total dose of 1.5–2 gm should be adequate for a true fungal pneumonia. The addition of 5-fluorocytosine may provide a more profound therapeutic effect, while surgical excision is usually recommended for a discrete fungus ball in the lung. In situations where the granulocyte count is rising, little or no treatment may be necessary.

Interstitial lung infiltrates in the febrile neutropenic patient are often caused by cytomegalovirus or *Pneumocystis carinii*. Cytomegalovirus (CMV) can be demonstrated by bronchoalveolar lavage, and either gancyclovir[6] or CMV immunoglobulin may be successful in treatment. Pneumocystis often induces dyspnea without visible changes on chest x-ray; alternatively, the chest x-ray may show hazy infiltrates spreading peripherally from the hila, and the breath sounds may be clear. The diagnosis is made by bronchoalveolar lavage or lung biopsy, though an empiric trial of trimethoprim-sulfamethoxazole is often warranted prior to a diagnostic procedure. Clinical improvement may not be evident for 4–5 days, and pentamidine is a useful adjunct in refractory cases (trimetrexate is a further alternative).

Infections of the central nervous system can be both dramatic and dangerous; *Cryptococcus* and *Listeria* are two of the most common infectious agents causing meningitis. The diagnosis of cryptococcal meningitis is confirmed by demonstrating specific antigen in the CSF (or serum), though an India Ink prep is positive in about 1/2 the cases. Preferred treatment is a combination of amphotericin B and oral 5-fluorocytosine. For *Listeria*, ampicillin or penicillin are both effective, though third generation cephalosporins are not.

Once an infection is suspected and a particular regimen is chosen, a variable period of close surveillance is necessary. Even if the source of infection is discovered, daily physical exams are necessary to detect any sequelae. If a patient does not improve within 72 hours of empiric therapy, it is appropriate to culture or biopsy any suspicious sites. Alternatively, one could add empiric erythromycin, trimethoprim-sulfamethoxazole, or vancomycin depending on the circumstances. If at any time a culture identifies a pathogen, the antibiotic schedule should be simplified as much as possible.

Patients considered at moderate risk are those whose fevers dissipate within 7 days and who experience a rising neutrophil count; once the absolute granulocyte count (including band forms) is ≥ 500, full recovery is likely. For those patients who do not have a recovery in granulocytes at 7 days, it is acceptable, if not prudent, to cover them for 14 days with a broad spectrum regimen. If the patient is also persistently febrile, one may add amphotericin B empirically after 7 days, since the likelihood of fungal superinfection increases at this point (ketoconazole may also be helpful as an alternative, though amphotericin B is required for any invasive fungal infection). If the patient is afebrile but still neutropenic at 14 days, stopping antibiotics may result in a 30% chance of a relapse with fever.[4]

Infections suspected to be related to indwelling venous access catheters represent a unique clinical situation and are discussed in Chapter 14. The majority of catheter related infections are due to staphylococci, and if coagulase-negative, a 10-day course of vancomycin should allow 80% of individuals to keep their catheters safely.[7] Antibiotic infusions should be rotated in each channel of a multi-channeled catheter. If an obvious tunnel infection is present, or cultures continue to be positive 24 hours after vancomycin has been started, the catheter should be removed. There appears to be no advantage to adding vancomycin at the outset in a neutropenic patient with fever and no obvious source;[8] vancomycin can be safely added when the culture results return.

In summary, consider the following steps once antibiotic treatment has started:

1. Monitor physical exam daily for evidence of progressive or secondary infection.
2. If cultures identify a pathogen, streamline antibiotic schedule.
3. If no improvement clinically at 72 hours, reculture or biopsy specific sites, or add supplementary antibiotic(s)—e.g. erythromycin, trimethoprim-sulfamethoxazole, vancomycin.
4. If no clinical improvement by day 7, empiric amphotericin B or ketoconazole may be added.
5. If absolute granulocyte count does not reach 500 by day 7, continue antibiotics until day 14.
6. If a coagulase-negative staphylococcus is isolated in a patient with a venous catheter, treat with vancomycin for 10 days and then reculture.
7. If a tunnel infection or persistently positive culture after 24 hours, catheter should be removed.
8. WASH HANDS BETWEEN PATIENTS.

Attempts to avoid infections in immunocompromised patients have not proved to be practically beneficial, even with specially equipped laminar airflow rooms and prophylactic antibiotics. Of note is the observation that less than 30% of physicians wash their hands between patients[9], yet this simple measure may be more protective than any other action.

BLEEDING IN THE CANCER PATIENT

Mild to moderate degrees of hemorrhage are rather commonplace in cancer patients, and fortunately serious bleeding is generally rare. Hemorrhage may be a direct consequence of tumor growth or a result of various indirect effects the neoplasm may engender. Primary tumors of the lung, colon, stomach, liver, and uterus will often present with variable amounts of bleeding, and if profuse enough, immediate surgery or radiation therapy will usually control the problem. More severe degrees of hemorrhage are seen late in the course of cancer when extensive tissue breakdown is accompanied by thrombocytopenia, liver or kidney dysfunction, and malnutrition.

Considering indirect effects, one of the most prominent predisposing factors for bleeding is thrombocytopenia. Frequently bone marrow replacement by tumor, splenomegaly, or treatment effects (chemotherapy and radiation) will render a patient thrombocytopenic during the course of his/her illness. An ITP-like syndrome has been described with certain lymphoproliferative tumors and carcinomas, characterized by a lack of anemia and no evidence for drug reaction or disseminated intravascular coagulation (DIC).[10] The treatment for this syndrome is an initial trial of corticosteroids (usually with mild success) and subsequent splenectomy.

Disseminated intravascular coagulation is a frequent cause of thrombocytopenia and may be seen as a complication of particular malignancies, including adenocarcinomas and acute promyelocytic leukemia. Manifestations of this condition range from no symptoms when it is in a compensated state (laboratory examination reveals elevated fibrin degradation products, increased or decreased fibrinogen levels, and mild clotting abnormalities) to frank thrombosis or hemorrhage. In a clinical setting where DIC is suspected, other etiologies such as sepsis, acidosis, hypotension, hypoxemia, and transfusion reaction should be ruled out. In an acute setting the treatment should primarily be directed at the underlying disease; if this is not totally feasible or successful, one should attempt to interrupt the major pathologic manifestation (heparin for thrombosis and clotting factors, platelets, whole blood with or without heparin in cases of hemorrhage).[11] Heparin is frequently used in induction therapy for acute promyelocytic leukemia, although it may be held until overt bleeding occurs or lab parameters change.[12] For chronic DIC heparin has been deemed successful in 2/3 of cases; a dose of 300–600 u/kg per 24 hours (either divided at 6–8 hour intervals or by continuous infusion) should be adequate.[13]

The general approach to thrombocytopenia is to alleviate the causative factor(s) sufficiently to allow for platelet recovery, but transfusion of platelets may be necessary at times to lower the risk of bleeding. A generally accepted principle is that platelet transfusions are warranted in *hypoproliferative situations* where levels drop below 20,000 per cu. mm. An expected rise of 6000–7000 platelets per unit of platelets transfused (or 48,000–50,000 per 8 unit pack) 1 hour after infusion is reasonable, unless active bleeding, splenomegaly, or fever are present. As transfused platelets typically last 3–4 days in the circulation, twice a week transfusions will usually keep the count greater than 20,000. If on two successive occasions the incremental rise after transfusion is 20% or less of predicted, the patient is considered refractory to platelet transfusions.[14] After 10–

25 transfusion episodes there is approximately a 25% chance of becoming refractory. In this setting HLA typing and appropriate matching of platelets should provide better results. If a patient develops an allergic reaction (urticaria) to a platelet transfusion, Benadryl is usually therapeutic; a febrile reaction with chills should respond to either acetaminophen, or demerol 0.5 mg/kg intravenously.

Qualitative platelet defects can also give rise to bleeding, as many commonly used medications inhibit platelet function (e.g. aspirin, ibuprofen). Certain antibiotics used frequently to treat infections in neutropenic patients (moxalactam, penicillin G, ticarcillin, piperacillin) can cause dysfunctional platelet aggregation, and moxalactam may cause hypoprothrombinemia. Recognition of these potential problems by checking a template bleeding time (for platelet dysfunction) and a protime (PT) plus partial thromboplastin time (PTT) is advised in appropriate settings. In addition, some B-lactam antibiotics, metranidazole, and sulfonamides may potentiate the effects of warfarin.[15]

MANAGEMENT OF NAUSEA AND VOMITING IN THE CANCER PATIENT

Nausea and vomiting in the cancer patient is a fairly common occurrence, resulting from either disease pathology or treatment side effects. Nausea is frequently a symptom that many associate with cancer, and is often dreaded by cancer patients. Although nausea and vomiting are anticipated side effects with many antineoplastic treatment regimens, these symptoms can be minimized with appropriate interventions. Management of nausea and vomiting is important not only for patient comfort and quality of life, but also to ensure compliance in continuing cancer therapy.

Although chemotherapy is the most common cause of nausea and vomiting in the cancer patient, there are additional etiologies related to the disease process or other treatments. Possible causes include hypercalcemia, bowel obstruction, liver metastasis, brain or leptomeningeal metastases, renal dysfunction, hypomagnesemia, narcotics and other medications, anxiety, and radiation therapy and immunotherapy effects. All possible causes of nausea and vomiting in the cancer patient must be addressed before appropriate management can be implemented.

The pathophysiology of vomiting is quite complex. The vomiting center in the lateral reticular formation of the medulla is responsible for initiating the act of vomiting, receiving stimuli from various parts of the body (see Figure 12.1).

Because of the many influencing factors, effective management of nausea and vomiting involves a variety of pharmacologic and nonpharmacologic interventions.

The exact mechanism of chemotherapy-induced emesis is unknown but is thought to be most closely related to the chemoreceptor trigger zone (CTZ). The CTZ is located on the floor of the fourth ventricle and is sensitive to noxious toxic substances circulating in the blood or cerebral spinal fluid (e.g. chemotherapy). Although in itself the CTZ does not cause vomiting, it does have the ability to stimulate the vomiting center through neural connection. The transmission of stimuli in the vicinity of the vomiting center and CTZ is thought to be mediated by neurotransmitters, such as dopamine, histamine, prostaglandins, serotonin, and acetylcholine. Therefore, many of the chemotherapy antiemetic programs include different agents that block these neurotransmitter sites.

The emetogenic potential varies among chemotherapeutic agents (see Table 12.1).

The specific chemotherapy program (intensity and location of administration), as well as the patient characteristics, will dictate the amount and types of antiemetics used. For programs that are moderately to

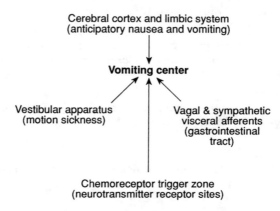

Figure 12.1   Pathophysiology of Vomiting

Table 12.1
Emetogenic Potential of Common Chemotherapeutic Agents

High	Moderate	Low
cisplatin	mitomycin-C	vinca alkaloids
mechlorethamine	doxorubicin (low dose)	5-fluorouracil
streptozotocin	cytarabine	etoposide
dacarbazine	procarbazine	bleomycin
cyclophosphamide (high dose)	methotrexate (high dose)	melphalan
daunorubicin	lomustine	methotrexate (low dose)
doxorubicin (moderate to high dose)	methyl-CCNU	L-asparaginase
	carboplatin mitoxantrone ifosfamide	chlorambucil

greatly emetogenic, or if the patient history suggests increased risk of emesis (motion sickness, bad previous experience with chemotherapy, high anxiety, or "vomiting-prone"), a combination of at least three antiemetics with different mechanisms of action should be administered prior to and after chemotherapy. Table 12.2 delineates the various antiemetics and routes of administration.

An example of a common combination of antiemetics used for an inpatient chemotherapy program of moderate or significant emetogenic potential includes:

A1. *Benzodiazapine*
   Lorazepam 0.5–2.0 mg. p.o. or IV one-half hour before chemotherapy, four to six hours after, every four hours prn.

and

2. *Corticosteroid*
   Dexamethasone 10–20 mg. IV one-half hour before and four hours after.

and

3. *Antihistamine*

Table 12.2
Antiemetic Agents—dosage, scheduling, and action

Phenothiazines

Prochlorperazine
Tablet (5, 10, 25 mg)	q. 4–6 hrs.	Dopamine antago-
Suppository (25 mg)	q. 6–8 hrs.	nist. Inhibits
Injection (5–10 mg)	q. 3–4 hrs.	vomiting center
IV or IM		by blocking auto-
		nomic afferents
		via vagus nerve

Perphenazine
Tablet 4 mg.	q. 4–6 hrs.	Dopamine antago-
Injection (5 mg) IV	q. 3–4 hrs.	nist. Inhibits
		vomiting center
		by blocking auto-
		nomic afferents
		via vagus nerve

Thiethylperazine maleate
Tablet (10 mg)	q. 4–6 hrs.	Dopamine antago-
Suppository (10 mg)	q. 4–6 hrs.	nist. Inhibits
Injection (10 mg)	q. 4–6 hrs.	vomiting center
		by blocking auto-
		nomic afferents
		via vagus nerve

Substituted Benzamides

Metoclopramide
Tablet (10 mg)	q. 4 hrs. (outpt.)	Dopamine antago- nist. Inhibits
Injection (1–2 mg/kg (IV)	30–60 min. prior to chemo., q. 2 hrs. for 4 doses	CTZ. Increases gastric emtpying

Benzodiazepines

Lorazepam
Tablet (0.5, 1, 2 mg)	30 min. prior to chemo., then q. 4–6 hrs. pm	CNS depressant. Anxiolytic seda- tive
Injection (0.5–2 mg) IV		

Table 12.2
Antiemetic Agents—dosage, scheduling, and action—continued

Glucocorticoids		
Dexamethasone		
Tablet (4 mg)	q. 4–6 hrs. 30	Unknown, may
Injection (10–20 mg) IV	min. prior to	act by inhibition
	chemo., then q. 4	of prostaglandins
	hrs. for 1–4	
	doses	
Prednisone		
Tablet (20 mg)	q. 6 hrs. prn	Unknown, may
	(outpt.)	act by inhibition
		of prostaglandins
Serotonin Antagonists		
Ondansetron		
IV (0.15 mg./kg.)	30 min. prior to	Selective
	chemotherapy,	antagonist of
	then q. 4 hrs. ×	seratonin S3
	2 after	receptors in GI
		tract and medulla
Cannabinoids		
Delta-9-tetrahydrocannabinol		
Tablets	q. 4 hrs. prn	Unknown, may
(5–10 mg/m^2)		act by CNS
		depression

Diphenhydramine 25–50 mg. IV one hour before, every four hours × 2 after, and every four hours prn.

and

4. *Phenothiazine*
Perphenazine 5 mg. IV *or* prochlorperazine 10–20 mg. IV one-half hour before, every four hours × 2 after, and every four hours prn.

or

5. *Substituted Benzamide*
Metoclopramide 1–2 mg./kg. IV one-half hour before, every two to four hours × 4 after, and every four hours prn.

Note: Due to similar toxicities, either a phenothiazine or metoclopramide is given, not both at the same time. *Extrapyramidal side effects* from phenothiazines and metoclopramide may occur and are more common with patients less than 40 years of age. Such symptoms include akathisia, neck dystonia, and oculogyric crisis, which are usually prevented or ameliorated with diphenhydramine or benztropine mesylate.

B1. *Serotonin Antagonist*
Ondansetron 0.15 mg./kg. IV one-half hour before, every four hours × 2 after

and

2. *Corticosteroid*
Dexamethasone 10–20 mg. IV one-half hour before and four hours after.

Recent investigations have provided promising results for the use of ondansetron in chemotherapy-related emesis. Ondansetron is a selective antagonist of serotonin S3 receptors, devoid of antidopaminergic properties. It blocks serotonin receptors both peripherally in the gastrointestinal tract as well as centrally in the medulla. It is very well tolerated and does not cause sedation or extrapyramidal side effects. The most common side effect is headache, occurring in approximately 14% of patients. For young patients less than 30 years of age who have a high tendency for extrapyramidal symptoms, or those who do not want to be sedated, ondansetron is especially useful. Efficacy is increased when administered in combination with dexamethasone.

Anticipatory symptoms occur when the thoughts, sights, smells, and sounds of the chemotherapy experience invoke nausea and vomiting prior to the actual chemotherapy administration. It is believed that this is due to stimulation of the vomiting center by the cerebral cortex and limbic system. Anxiety seems to be a significant contributing factor; therefore, by minimizing prechemotherapy anxiety (up to 48 hours before) by either anxiolytics and behavioral relaxation techniques, anticipatory nausea and vomiting may be decreased. Also, patients that have had a poor prior experience with chemotherapy are more likely to experience anticipatory symptoms.

Delayed nausea and vomiting occur beginning twenty-four hours or more after chemotherapy administration. Although this may occur with different chemotherapy drugs, it is most common with moderate to high doses of cisplatin or doxorubicin. To prevent or treat delayed emesis, maintain the patient on regular doses of antiemetics up to four days after chemotherapy administration (e.g. dexamethasone 2–4 mg. p.o. twice a day, and metoclopramide 20 mg. p.o. four times a day).

CANCER-RELATED PAIN

Although the total number of patients with cancer-related pain accounts for only five percent of the chronic pain population,[16] cancer pain afflicts nearly 800,000 Americans and some eighteen million patients worldwide per year. It is undeniably a major clinical problem as fifty to eighty percent of patients with metastatic disease experience pain.[18,19,20]

I. Pain Syndromes

Pain syndromes that develop in cancer patients can be divided into five major groups: a) those caused by direct tumor involvement; b) those associated with cancer therapy; c) those due to the debilitating effects of the disease; d) those totally unrelated to the cancer; and e) a combination of two or more of these types.[17,18]

A. Tumor Involvement

Cancer pain associated with direct tumor involvement may be caused by bone invasion, nerve compression or infiltration, spinal cord compression, visceral invasion, blood vessel infiltration, or mucous membrane inflammation/necrosis (see Table 12.3).

B. *Treatment-Related*

1. *Surgery*

In a small percentage of patients who undergo thoracotomy, postsurgical pain is present. Pain in the distribution of an intercostal nerve becomes evident within one or two months following the surgical procedure. Movement exacerbates the pain, and these patients may develop concomitant frozen shoulder characterized by limitation of movement at the shoulder joint and disuse atrophy of the arm.

Pain in the posterior arm, axilla, and anterior chest wall in patients following radical mastectomy occurs due to interruption of the intercostobrachial nerve, a cutaneous branch of T1 nerves. This tight, constricting, burning pain may occur one to two months after surgery and is more common in patients with a complicated post-operative course of either excessive local swelling or infection. Due to an exacerbation of pain by arm

Table 12.3
Types of Cancer Pain Related to Direct Tumor Involvement

Type of Tumor Involvement	Location of Pain	Description of Pain
Bone invasion	Localized or referred	Constant and progressive
Nerve compression or infiltration	Areas of affected nerve plexus	Burning, shooting, and constant
Spinal cord compression	Back	Dull, aching severe, radicular
Visceral invasion	Referred to related dermatomes	Diffuse, poorly localized
Blood vessel infiltration	Usually localized to affected limb or part of body	Burning, aching, and diffuse
Mucous membrane inflammation, ulceration, or necrosis	Localized	Burning and excruciating

movement, a frozen shoulder may develop as occurs in post-thoracotomy pain syndromes.

A number of patients who undergo radical neck dissection develop a constant burning sensation, dysesthesias, and intermittent shock-like pain in the neck from interruption of the cervical nerves. Following amputation of a limb, the patients may develop pain in the stump and/or in the phantom limb. Stump pain is usually constant and burning in character, whereas pain in the phantom limb may be either burning or cramping such as might be caused by abnormal positioning of the distal part of a limb.

2. Chemotherapy

Post-chemotherapy pain may occur following treatment with the Vinca alkaloid drugs. A symmetrical polyneuropathy, characterized by burning pain exacerbated by superficial stimuli, is commonly localized to the hands and feet.

Steroid pseudo-rheumatism occurs from withdrawal of steroid medications in patients taking these drugs for either short or long periods of time. The syndrome consists of prominent diffuse myalgia and arthralgia, with muscle and joint tenderness on palpation, but without objective inflammatory signs. These signs and symptoms revert with reinstitution of the steroid medication.

Necrosis of the head of the femur and/or humerus occurs as a complication of chronic steroid therapy in cancer patients, most commonly with Hodgkin's disease. The pain is often the presenting symptom and is characterized by deep, dull, constant and severe aching in the knee and shoulder joint. These patients experience limitation of joint movement and a progressive inability to use the arm.

Mucositis occurs in the mouth, throat, nasal passages, and gastrointestinal tract as a result of toxicity from various chemotherapeutic agents. A consequence of sloughing of mucous membranes is an excruciating pain that interferes with eating, drinking, and possibly talking.

3. Radiation Therapy

Pain occurring in the distribution of the brachial plexus following radiation therapy results from fibrosis of the surrounding connective tissue and secondary to nerve injury. It may appear as early as six months or as late as twenty years following radiation treatments, and represents a difficult diagnostic problem in that it must be differentiated from recurrent tumor. Initial symptoms include numbness and paresthesias in the hand. Diffuse arm pain, lymphedema, and neurologic signs of motor weakness and sensory changes in the C5,6,7 distribution are later symptoms.

Radiation fibrosis of the lumbar plexus represents a similar diagnostic problem of radiation injury versus recurrent tumor. Progressive motor and sensory changes in the leg followed by leg pain are consistent with radiation fibrosis.

As a result of spinal cord irradiation, radiation myelopathy may occur which results in pain and neurologic changes. The pain may be localized to the area of spinal-cord damage or may be referred pain, with dysesthesias below the level of injury. Clinically, the neurologic symptoms and signs are those of a

Brown-Sequard syndrome: ipsilateral motor paresis and contralateral sensory loss at a cervical or thoracic level, which progresses to a complete transverse myelopathy.

C. Debilitating Effects of Cancer

There are a variety of negative effects, including pain, that the cancer patient experiences as a result of debilitation from the cancer and/or the treatment. For example, many patients in the terminal stages of their disease become weak, dehydrated,and eventually bedbound; this, in turn, may result in bed sores which contribute to the pre-existing pain. The combination of inactivity, poor p.o. intake, and administration of narcotics causes constipation, which adds to a cancer patient's discomfort. Also, emotional stress and impaired activity level may contribute to muscle tension/spasms and myofascial pain symdromes.

Due to altered immune states that result from chemotherapy, radiation therapy, or the disease process, cancer patients are prone to infections which may lead to other sites of pain. Infected skin ulcerations or lacerations can be inflamed and extremely tender. Urinary tract infections result in urgency, frequency, and dysuria. Rectal abcesses pose excruciating discomfort and difficulty with defecation. Other infections may also occur affecting any or all body systems, compounding the level and complexity of pain.

D. Unrelated to Cancer

Approximately three percent of the pain syndromes which occur in cancer patients have no relationship to the underlying cancer or cancer therapy.[18] Degenerative disc disease, thoracic and abdominal aneurysms, migraine headaches, and diffuse osteoporosis are the most common non-cancer pain syndromes observed.

E. Combination of Pain Syndromes

There are numerous combinations of pain sydromes that may occur. An example of such a combination is post-herpetic neuralgia. The true incidence of this clinical entity is unknown, but appears to be more common in patients who develop the herpes zoster infection after the age of 50, and possibly a greater incidence in lymphoma patients. The herpes zoster infection commonly occurs in an area of tumor pathology or in the port of previous irradiation, and is characterized by pain which persists after the clearing of cutaneous eruptions from the herpes zoster infection.

II. Pain Management

    A. Pharmacologic (see Table 12.4)

        1. Non-Narcotics

            Aspirin, acetaminophen, and the family of non-steroidal anti-inflammatory drugs play an important role in cancer pain management. These drugs inhibit the synthesis of prostaglandin, both peripherally and centrally. The presumed mechanism of action is the inhibition of the enzyme cyclooxygenase, preventing formation of prostaglandin E2.[21] In addition to this action,

Table 12.4
Analgesic Agents

Drug	Dosage	Duration	Comments
Aspirin	650 mg.	4–6 hrs.	Platelet effects and gastric irritation makes uses limited
Acetaminophen	650 mg.	4–6 hrs.	Less anti-inflammatory activity
Ibuprofen	400–800 mg.	4–6 hrs.	Helpful for bone pain
Morphine	Oral 30–60 mg. IM 10 mg.	3–4 hrs.	Sustained release tablets last 8–12 hrs.
Oxycodone	Oral 10 mg.	4 hrs.	Often combined with aspirin or acetaminophen
Codeine	Oral 30–60 mg. IM 130 mg.	3–4 hrs. 3–4 hrs.	Also used in combinations
Hydromorphone	Oral 2–4 mg.	4 hrs.	Effective alternative
Levorphanol	Oral 2–4 mg. SC 2 mg.	4–5 hrs. 4–5 hrs.	Longer acting than most
Meperidine	Oral 50–150 mg. IM 75 mg.	2–4 hrs. 2–4 hrs.	CNS hyperirritability a concern
Methadone	Oral 5–20 mg. IM 5–20 mg.	5–6 hrs. 5–6 hrs.	May accumulate causing sedation

aspirin and non-steroidal anti-inflammatory drugs decrease the inflammatory reaction at the site of tumor or tissue injury. Also, these drugs may act synergistically with narcotic analgesics, which modulate pain in the central nervous system. This co-analgesic effect during concomitant narcotic administration may result in better pain control with fewer side effects. When used independently, these agents are effective for mild to moderate pain.

Other drugs which are commonly used for other purposes play a role in the management of cancer-related pain. For example, low to moderate dosages of tricyclic antidepressants as well as anticonvulsants are helpful adjuncts in the management of neurogenic pain. In addition, steroid therapy is quite beneficial for a variety of cancer pain syndromes, including soft tissue infiltration, nerve compression, visceral distention, lymphedema, increased intracranial pressure, and certain bone metastases (e.g. prostate carcinoma).

2. Narcotics (see Table 12.5)

Binding sites or receptors for opiate drugs are found at several places in the brain and spinal cord, as well as other tissues. The narcotic agonists relieve pain by binding to these specific receptors. The periaqueductal grey (PAG) area of upper brainstem appears to be the major site of narcotic action.

Morphine is the most common and most effective drug for chronic cancer pain. The vast majority of patients with moderate to severe chronic pain can be controlled on a regular schedule of oral morphine, which is available in long-acting tablets.

Hydromorphone is a potent, safe, and effective narcotic agent that is a derivative of morphine. It is essentially interchangeable with morphine in its value for patients with advanced cancer. It is more soluble than morphine and is relatively short-acting, with three to four hours' duration.

Methadone is an effective narcotic agent with a pharmacological action similar to morphine. Its advantages are that it is non-cross reactive with morphine in the face of a true morphine allergy, and it is much less expensive than equianalgesic doses of morphine or hydromorphone. One major concern with the use of methadone is accumulation. The pharmacokinetics of

Table 12.5
Narcotic Dose Equivalents for the Control of Chronic Pain[22]

Oral (P.O.) Dose (mg)[a]	Analgesic[b]	Subcutaneous (S.C.) Dose (mg.)
150	Meperidine (Demerol)[c]	50
100	Codeine[c] (Tylenol #3)	60
90	Pentazocine (Talwin)	30
15	Morphine (Roxanol, MSIR, MS Contin)[d,e]	5
10	Oxycodone (Percodan, Percocet, Tylox)[f]	7.5
10	Methadone (Dolophine)[g]	5
5	Oxymorphone (Numorphan)[h]	1
4	Hydromorphone (Dilaudid)[e]	1.5
2	Levorphanol (Levo-dromoran)	1

[a]*Equianalgesic doses* listed were obtained from a variety of sometimes conflicting studies and experiences and are meant only as guidelines for "by-the-clock", standing order analgesic therapy of chronic pain. No analgesic listed is superior p.o. to its equianalgesic dose of p.o. morphine.
[b]*Dose interval*: Every 3–4 hours for all except:
meperidine = q2–3h, levorphanol = q4–6h, methadone = q6–8h, MS Contin = q12h.
[c]Of little value in severe chronic pain.
[d]Equianalgesic *intravenous (i.v.)* dose = 3–4 mg q3–4h.
[e]*Rectal suppositories* available. Per rectum (p.r.) dose is equal to p.o. dose. *Subcutaneous (s.c.)* dose essentially equal to intramuscular (i.m.) dose.
[f]Oxycodone 10 mg = 2 Percodan, 2 Percocet, or 2 Tylox.
[g]*Caution*: Sedative side effects often accumulate despite inadequate analgesic effect.
[h]Available for non-parenteral use in rectal suppository form only.

methadone are complex, with the analgesic action lasting four to eight hours and the serum half-life being approximately twenty-five hours. Due to the propensity of patients and clinicians to give methadone on a more frequent basis or increase its dose more frequently that its half-life would safely allow, it is common to see methadone patients oversedated yet still in pain.

For mild to moderate pain, codeine and oxycodone are effective narcotic analgesics. Oxycodone is frequently administered in combination with acetaminophen or aspirin. Codeine, although a safe and effective agent, if administered at a dose equivalent to 15 mg. of morphine (100 mg. of codeine), causes considerably more gastrointestinal and neuropsychiatric effects.

Meperidine has a chemical structure that is quite different from that of morphine, but which binds to the opioid receptors to produce essentially the same type of analgesic effect. Meperidine is widely used in acute and post-operative pain partially because of its decreased spasmogenic effect on smooth muscle. However, in chronic cancer pain it is a poor analgesic choice since its' duration of action is short (two to three hours); it has low analgesic potency when given by mouth; and it may produce central nervous system excitation or convulsions with repeated large doses, due to accumulation of a toxic metabolite, normeperidine. Merperidine, in this patient population, is only for those who have a true allergy to morphine and cannot tolerate methadone.

B. Non-pharmacologic

Non-pharmacologic pain interventions can be beneficial adjuncts to the patient with cancer pain. Behavioral therapy, including distraction, imagery, and hypnosis, diminishes pain perception through central mechanisms. Progressive muscle relaxation and massage therapy both decrease muscle tension, as well as provide for positive distractions. Transcutaneous electrical stimulation (TENS) may also provide pain relief. Lastly, the use of both ice and heat is effective, although variable, in alleviating some forms of cancer-related pain.

GUIDELINES FOR MANAGEMENT OF PAIN IN THE CANCER PATIENT

1. *Comprehensive pain evaluation.*
   * Assess the site, quality, intensity, onset and duration, and factors that influence the pain.
   * In addition to complete initial assessments, frequent follow-up reassessments are important to check for response to pain therapy and possible tolerance.

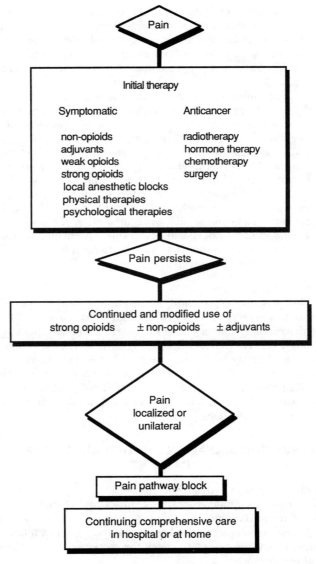

Figure 12.2

* Many cancer patients have more than one pain—each pain needs individual attention.
* Always trust the patient's description of his/her pain.
2. *Choose appropriate drug or drug combinations by individualizing to patient's specific pain.*
   * Know the pharmacology of the drug, including the duration of analgesic effect, pharmacokinetic properties, and equianalgesic doses.
3. *Adjust route of administration to patient's needs.*
4. *Administer on a scheduled (around-the-clock), rather than an as needed (prn) basis.*
5. *Individually titrate dose.*
   * There is no set optimal or maximal dose.
   * The right dose is that which controls pain without excessive or intolerable side effects.
6. *Tolerance will occur in all patients that chronically take narcotics.*
   * To overcome tolerance, increasing the dosage or frequency of administration of the narcotic is necessary to control pain.
   * An alternative is to switch to another narcotic drug by using one-half the equianalgesic dose as the starting dose, and slowly escalating the dose.
7. *Taper narcotics slowly.*
   * Abrupt discontinuation of narcotics in a patient that has been chronically taking them will produce withdrawal symptomatology such as agitation, tremors, insomnia, fever, and marked excitability of the autonomic nervous system.
   * To suppress narcotic withdrawal symptoms, reinstitute the drug at approximately 25% of the previous daily dose.
8. *Anticipate, prevent, and treat narcotic side effects.*
   * Bowel prep should be maintained, including stool softener and laxatives; as dosage of narcotics increases, a more aggressive bowel regimen is necessary.
   * Nausea and vomiting can be minimized by the use of antiemetics.
   * Excess sedation may be reduced, while sustaining pain relief, by decreasing individual doses and increasing the frequency of administration; in addition, amphetamines may be useful for some patients.
   * Respiratory depression in the tolerant patient can be reversed by the administration of the opioid antagonist naloxone (diluted 0.4 mg. in 10 cc. normal saline and titrated carefully).
9. *Respect each patient and accept individual differences.*

  * Analgesic response and side effects vary.
  * All complaints must be respected and addressed, such that pain control is maximized and side effects are minimized.
10. *Address the various factors that may influence the patient's pain—psychological, social, spiritual, and financial.*
  * Intervene appropriately and make referrals as necessary.
11. *Utilize nonpharmacologic interventions for pain control, including behavioral and/or physical therapies.*
12. *Remember, addiction and tolerance are not clinical problems in the patient with metastatic cancer—the patient and family may need reassurance about this issue.*

REFERENCES

1. Pizzo, P.A., Commers, J., Cotton, D. Approaching the controversies in antibacterial management of cancer patients. *Am J Med* 76:436, 1984.
2. Nelson, S., Chidiac, C., Summer, W. New strategies for preventing nosocomial pneumonia. *J Crit Illness* 3:12, 1988.
3. Magnussen, C.R. The new penicillins: pros and cons for serious infections. *J Crit Illness* 2:57, 1987.
4. Pizzo, P.A., Meyers, J. Infections in the cancer Patient. In DeVita, V.T., Hellman S., Rosenberg, S.A. (eds.) Cancer-Principles and Practice of Oncology (3rd ed.), J.B. Lippincott Company, Philadelphia, 1989, p. 2088–2127.
5. Pagani, J.J., Libshitz, H.I. Opportunistic fungal pneumonias in cancer patients. *Am J Rad* 137:1033, 1989.
6. Erice, A., Jordan, M.C., Chase, B.A., et al. Gancyclovir treatment of cytomegalovirus disease in transplant recipients and other immunocompromised hosts. *JAMA* 257:3082, 1987.
7. Pizzo, P.A. Diagnosis and management of infectious disease problems in the child with malignant disease. In Rubin, R.H., and Young, L.S. Clinical Approaches to the Infections in the Compromised Host. Plenum Publishing, New York, 1988, p. 439–464.
8. Rubin, M., Todeschini G., Marshall, D. et al. Does the presence of an indwelling venous catheter affect the type of infections in neutropenic cancer patients? An analysis of 505 episodes. Interscience Conference on Antimicrobial Agents and Chemotherapy, New York, 1987, p. 264.
9. Albert, R.K., Condie, F. Handwashing patterns in medical intensive care units. *N Engl J Med* 304:1465, 1981.
10. Kim, H.D., Boggs, D.R. A syndrome resembling idiopathic thrombocytopenic purpura in 10 patients with diverse forms of cancer. *Am J Med* 67:371, 1979.
11. Colman, R.W., Robboy, S.J., Minna, J.D. Disseminated intravascular coagulation: A reappraisal. *Annu Rev Med* 30:359, 1979.

12. Goldberg, M.A., Ginsberg, D., Mayer, R.J., et al. Is heparin administration necessary during induction chemotherapy for patients with acute promyelocytic leukemia? *Blood* 69:187, 1987.
13. Bunn, P.A., Ridgway, E.C. Paraneoplastic syndromes. In DeVita, V.T., Hellman, S., Rosenberg, S.A. (eds) *Cancer-Principles and Practices of Oncology*, J.B. Lippincott Company, Philadelphia, 1989, p. 1896–1933.
14. Reich, L.M., Dinsmore, R.E. Platelet transfusions: when and why? *Prim Care and Cancer*, 6:1(OR) 1986.
15. Hochman, R., Clark, J., Rolla, A., et al. Bleeding in patients with infections: Are antibiotics helping or hurting? *Arch Intern Med* 142:1440, 1982.
16. Bonica, J.J. Advances in pain research and therapy, Vol. 9, Raven Press, New York, 1985.
17. Benedetti, C., and Bonica, J.J. Advances in Pain Research and Therapy, Vol. 7, Raven Press, New York., 1984.
18. Foley, K.M. Advances in Pain Research and Therapy, Vol. 2 Raven Press, New York, 1985.
19. Daut, R.L. and Cleeland, C.S. The prevalence and severity of pain in cancer. *Cancer* 50:1913–1918, 1982.
20. Ahles, T.A., Ruckdeschel, J.C., and Blanchard, E.B. Cancer related pain— I. Prevalence in an outpatient setting as a function of stage of disease and type of cancer. *J Psychosom Res.* 28:115–119, 1984.
21. World Health Organization *Cancer pain relief*, World Health Organization, Geneva, Switzerland, 1986.
22. Levy, M.H. Pain management in advanced cancer. *Semin in Oncoll.* 12:394–410, 1985.

Chapter 13

Ethical Issues in Oncology Care

INTRODUCTION

The contemporary house officer faces many ethical issues in the care of the oncology patient. In an informal survey of medical interns at an acute care hospital, it was noted that they spend 30–60 percent of their time dealing with psychosocial, placement, and ethical issues. Cancer patients are the focus of many of the ethical dilemmas. The house officer must interact with the patient from the initial work-up leading to the diagnosis, through the treatment period, and possibly the patient's death, facing ethical issues at every step. *Responding appropriately to the ethical issues is an important aspect of the house officer's role.*

It is the house officer's responsibility, in conjunction with the oncologist, to make an accurate diagnosis and prognosis, to recommend appropriate therapies, and to communicate skillfully with the patient. The house officer's and patient's (or family member's) ethical values guide the related decision-making. At one time, it was held that physicians directed all the patient care and made decisions about treatments, and it was the patient's role to comply. *Today, based on moral and legal thinking, the patient, or the representatives of incompetent patients, can choose to accept or refuse treatments.*[1] This is a fundamental issue for medical ethics and the physician-patient relationship. *The house officer should promote the patient's health and well-being in accordance with the patient's desires.* This shared decision-making process is based on the moral rule of respect for the individual's self-determination or "do not deprive freedom."[2] *The physician should offer what he/she believes will be of benefit, and the patient is free to accept or refuse.*

VALID CONSENT OR REFUSAL

The concept of valid consent and refusal is the foundation for the practice of ethical medical care. In fact, there are very few ethical dilemmas that do not involve the concept. Valid consent is mandated both ethically and legally. Patient preferences are always important, but particularly so with the cancer patient, because the treatments frequently offer only minimum benefits and the refusal of the treatments is quite reasonable. Also, since many patients may eventually become terminally ill, they should be cared for in the manner they desire. In seeking to know and in respecting the patient's desires, the house officer is accepting the ethical significance of self-determination, a basic moral rule.

Underlying this line of thinking is the assumption that the house officer or another member of the medical team has told the patient about the presence of cancer. Patients need to be told the truth about their situation in a caring and supportive manner as soon as the diagnosis is established. The physician should communicate the information in a private and comfortable environment using understandable language, indicating that appropriate treatments will be discussed (offering hope), and the patient and family (when present) should be given an opportunity to ask questions and express their feelings about the diagnosis. Open communication strengthens the physician-patient relationship, promotes moral integrity, and can improve the consent process.

There are three basic requirements for a valid consent or refusal.[3] *First, patients must receive adequate information about the tests, procedures, and treatments offered to them.* Adequate information includes the risks and benefits associated with the suggested treatment, any rea-

---

**Valid consent
or refusal:**

- Adequate information

- No coercion

- Competence

sonable alternative treatment(s), and the option of no treatment at all. Besides understanding the possible benefit of the treatment, patients need to know about the relevant risks, including death, pain (both physical and psychological), disability, and loss of freedom. Reasonable alternative treatments should be presented to the patient in an unbiased manner. It is also very important for patients to understand the probable outcome of having no treatment. This is particularly important for cancer patients, because the treatments can be so uncertain and difficult that "no treatment," except for supportive care, is a reasonable option.

I have emphasized the importance of providing full information, but occasionally patients say, "I do not want all that information," and want the physician to make the decision. House officers should be reluctant to take on this role, because medical decision-making is a personal value decision based on the patient's assessment of quality and quantity of life and sense of purpose and meaning in life. It is the physician's role to make a decision regarding the treatment options. However, it is the patient's decision to accept or refuse the treatment based on their values as to what is best for them. There are some patients who insist on not wanting to make the decision. *If the competent patient explicitly does not want to know the risks and benefits and wants you to make the decision, it is morally permissible for the house officer to do so.* The house officer is not required to do so. Such decision-making may require review by the attending physician, depending on the particular hospital's policy. Even if the house officer does make the treatment decision, they should share the decision with the patient giving them the opportunity to respond to that decision.

A second component of a valid consent is no coercion. A house officer is free to recommend a treatment but should not force the patient with strong negative incentives that make it unreasonable for the patient to resist. Physicians can strongly recommend a treatment, yet patients should clearly understand that they are the ones making the final decision.

Thirdly, for consent or refusal to be valid, the patient must be competent. Competence is a legal term but not exclusively used within the courts. For physicians, it refers to the ability to make a particular decision. In caring for cancer patients, as well as others, it is best to think of the capacity to make decisions in regard to the particular decision being discussed. A person is or is not competent to make the particular decision. Therefore, a patient may be able to appreciate and understand one particular decision, but not another decision. For example, patients may be competent to decide what they want for lunch but unable to choose between chemotherapy and no treatment. The capacity to make health care decisions rests on the patient's ability to appreciate and understand the information that is being presented in the consent process and recognizing they are being asked to choose between the options. Competency is the ability to make a decision. You should know whether patients are competent or not prior to their making actual decisions. Competency is not determined by the quality of their decision or whether they are willing to accept the recommended treatment.

Caring for cancer patients forces the physician to realize that there are three levels of the capacity to make decisions: incompetent, partially competent, and fully competent.[4] Incompetent patients may be comatose and completely unaware of their surroundings, or they may have limited cognitive abilities (for example, be able to recognize someone's face or yell out for water if thirsty) but still be unable to understand the consent process. If one does suggest a treatment to such a patient, the patient either cannot answer or answers in some random fashion. These patients have no degree of understanding or appreciation.

Partially competent cancer patients can give a simple consent or refusal, but not a valid consent or valid refusal. These patients understand that they are being asked to consent or refuse, and they do consent or refuse, but they lack the ability to understand and appreciate adequately the information conveyed to them during the consent process. They can only give consent or refusal to a decision that requires minimum understanding. However, a decision that requires only a minimum amount of understanding, such as whether one wants a hamburger or a salad for lunch, can be a valid decision for such a patient.

Patients with cancer fall into this category frequently. An example of partial competence would be a very ill patient with widespread metastatic disease who agrees to be treated with a systemic chemotherapeutic agent but who cannot repeat or remember most of the information provided during the consent process about the unpleasant side effects expected from the drug. This patient has consented, but the quality of consent is badly compromised: the patient understands little of the information and may not even know that it applies to him or her. The patient's consent cannot be considered valid, and a proxy decision-maker should be sought. Equally, if the patient refuses treatment a proxy decision-maker should be sought. This situation is complicated when the partially competent patient refuses and the proxy consents because the patient's cooperation is necessary for most treatments. When the patient is clearly not cooperative, a review of the decision is essential to evaluate whether the potential benefits of the treatment are so great that they outweigh the evils of forced treatment.

The overwhelming majority of patients are competent to give a valid consent or a valid refusal. They are fully competent: they understand the information given to them during the consent process, and they appreciate that it applies to them at this point in time. If the potential benefits are so great and the evils or harms are minimal, the house officer is justified to treat the unwilling patient.[4]

I have presented three criteria for a valid consent, yet *it is important to note that the requirements for a patient to consent to a treatment are the same requirements for refusing a treatment.* A patient who gives a valid refusal must receive adequate information, must not be coerced, and must be competent.

There is a legal parallel to the ethical basis for valid consent or refusal. Frequently, the law and ethics seem to be at odds with one another. However, regarding valid consent or refusal there is general consensus. Many judicial decisions and laws support the ethical concept that an adult person can choose or refuse treatments and that a consent process must be employed.

LOCUS OF DECISION-MAKING

Many of the moral problems faced by house officers involve cancer patients in the end stages of life. The decisions concerning the endpoint of health care can be difficult and emotionally painful for both the patient, family, and house officer. This is especially true if the house officer limits his role to that of curing the patient. A more accurate perception is for the physician to see his or her role as promoting the health and well-being of the patient for as long as possible according to the patient's desires. This may include the patient's desire to die sooner rather than later. The house officer is to help such patients facilitate their goals, values, and sense of meaning.[5]

The house officer should openly discuss with competent patients their goals and desires. Often, however, the more difficult ethical cases house officers confront do not involve the fully competent patient. When a patient is no longer competent to consent or refuse treatment, the physician should try to identify and follow the previously stated preferences of the patient. *An advance directive is a document or oral statement given by a competent patient to direct the extent and level of care desired in the event the patient is incompetent.*[6] A common example of an advance directive is a Do-Not-Resuscitate order, including no CPR, intubation, or ventilation. Advance directives can be extremely helpful and should be routinely sought, especially for terminally ill or chronically ill cancer patients. Conversations with patients about what they would or would not desire are generally welcomed by patients because they serve as a means of facilitating self-determination and control.[7] The physician should be able to anticipate potential problems in addition to resuscitation because of the physician's understanding of the natural history of the disease process. For example, the house officer should discuss with "end stage" lung cancer patients whether or not they would want antibiotics in the event of pneumonia and clearly document the patient's wishes. House officers should serve as consultants engaged to evaluate their patient's present problem and future problems and present all reasonable options for treatment in understandable language, and foster optimal patient decision-making.[8]

In many hospitals, only the attending can write orders to limit therapy, but the house officer can help create the environment for good communication with the patient by helping them to understand their prognosis and potential future health care needs. This may take time for the busy and often sleep-deprived house officer, but *a clear understanding of what the patient would or would not want if or when they are incapable of making decisions can save time and stress, and can reduce ethical dilemmas in the long run.*

One of the most frequently used advance directives is the Living Will. This is a legally nonbinding document in its generic form but, in the majority of states, a legally binding document when properly executed under the "Terminal Care Document" or "Natural Death Act" statutes. Any competent adult can sign such a document, which indicates that when a person is incompetent, terminally ill, and there is no reasonable expectation of recovery, he/she does not want to be kept alive by heroic or extraordinary measures.

A *Living Will* is a welcome improvement compared to not knowing what an incompetent patient would desire. The document should be placed in the patient's chart. However, because of the vagueness of the language and the narrow focus on only terminal situations, the Living Will may have limited usefulness and it can even create problems. The Living Will succeeds in providing a general idea of the patient's wishes but fails to provide the detailed instructions necessary for the physician. In these cases, the physician faces the unenviable task of having to make his or her own interpretation of the vague provisions of the Living Will. There is the obvious possibility that the physician may inadvertently misinterpret the patient's wishes and provide a level of care that may be more aggressive or less aggressive than that which the patient intended. Even with these problems the Living Will, when properly executed in those states where legally authorized, grants physicians civil and criminal immunity if they follow what they believe to be the patient's intended desires.

A more flexible directive is the *Durable Power of Attorney for Health Care (DPAHC). The DPAHC permits an adult to designate a person (agent) who is authorized to make surrogate medical decisions when the patient becomes incompetent.*[4,6] Many states now have DPAHC statutes that provide legal authority for such a designation. The main benefit of the DPAHC provision is its flexibility to adapt the patient's value system to any particular clinical situation through the decision of the surrogate.

Physicians should encourage patients to make their Living Will or DPAHC provisions as specific as possible. When presented with a Living Will, physicians should discuss what the document means to the patient and how it should be applied to the situations relevant to the patient's health status. This information should be placed in the chart along with the document. The agent designated by the DPAHC should be familiar with the patient and should be instructed regarding their specific preferences. In our overly litigious society the use of a Living Will and DPAHC can be helpful rather than just having verbal understanding with the patient. Even if a formal DPAHC is not used, *the house officer should ask the competent patient to indicate who they would like to make decisions for them in the event they are incapable of making decisions for themselves. This is particularly important if the house officer is aware:*

• That there are any family conflicts;
• That there is no family;

- That there is any uncertainty about who (within large families) should serve as the patient's proxy;
- That the only visitor is a non-relative; or
- That the "ex-spouse" is still legally married to the patient.

Clarifying the issue while the patient is competent will decrease future (time consuming) problems. The person identified as the surrogate decision-maker should be notified by the patient if possible or by a member of the health care team. The house officer should document who is the designated person in the patient's chart and where they can be reached.

In the absence of a clear and documented advance directive, a proxy or surrogate decision maker should be sought. *The proxy should be asked to express the decision the patient would have made in the particular situation rather than the decision the surrogate would personally choose.* This process is referred to as the doctrine of substituted judgment.[5,9] The surrogate can be either the agent designated by the DPAHC or a court-appointed guardian for health care decision-making. If there is such a legally designated surrogate, the physician should respect this surrogate's valid consent or refusal.

When there is no legally appointed surrogate, the physician should turn to the next-of-kin. Although next-of-kin may lack legal authority, following their decisions is morally appropriate because they can provide substitute judgment. Physicians have the responsibility to provide the surrogate with adequate information without coercion to optimize their decision-making ability. House officers can reduce the guilt the proxy may feel by reassuring them that the decision is the one that the patient would have made.

A less attractive level of decision-making is in the concept of best interest, i.e., in the absence of clear guidance from the patient, someone, usually the next of kin, is asked to express what they believe to be in the patient's best overall interest. The difference in this level of decision-making is the absence of clear and specific guidance from the patient to the physician or the proxy. The ethical validity of decisions based on the proxy's subjective perception of the patient's best interest is problematic. Surrogates who do not know the patient's preferences apply the best interest standard, considering issues such as cultural or religiously shared values, perceived beliefs, degree of suffering, and quality of life with and without the treatment.[10] Even though this level of decision-making has the potential for problems, it can be commonly applied in the clinical setting because the surrogate knows the patient best, the decision seems reasonable, the decisionmaker does not appear to have any hidden agenda, and the decision is not inconsistent with what the health care providers know about the patient.

The last level of decision-making is the situation in which there is no representative for the patient. If the situation is not an emergency, a court appointed guardian should be obtained. In many states this is a long process. *House Officers need to be aware of their particular hospital's policy, but the point is clear—try to avoid the long court appointed process by seeking clear directives from the patient during the planning of the patient's management.*

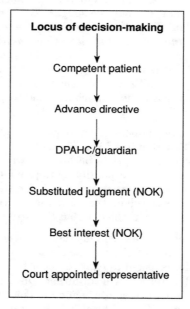

Locus of decision-making

Competent patient

Advance directive

DPAHC/guardian

Substituted judgment (NOK)

Best interest (NOK)

Court appointed representative

SOME DIFFICULT CLINICAL DISTINCTIONS

In making medical decisions for end-stage cancer patients, there are several common distinctions frequently discussed that need to be clarified.

Withholding vs. Withdrawing Treatment

Some physicians feel that under certain circumstances it may be appropriate to withhold therapy, but that therapies cannot be withdrawn once started. This distinction is not ethically justified. The reason to start a treatment is based on its potential benefits and the patient's consent. If the actual benefits are much less or the risks are much greater than anticipated, and the competent patient offers a rational refusal of treatment, the treatment should be discontinued. In this line of thinking it is actually easier to determine whether or not it is medically appropriate to discontinue a treatment because of the specific understanding of the treatment's benefit compared to general knowledge about the treatment when it was proposed. The real difference between withholding and withdrawing is more psychological than ethical.[8]

This issue can be a part of the advance directive decision. For example, a lung cancer patient receiving chemotherapy may consent to full resuscitation including ventilation but indicate that they would want the ventilator removed if after a few days it becomes clear that the patient's compromised lungs will not allow him or her to be weaned from the ventilator. Such a decision is morally valid and promotes good medical care.

Ordinary vs. Extraordinary Treatment

Another commonly used distinction in considering the treatments for cancer patients is whether they are ordinary or extraordinary. If a treatment is extraordinary, it may be withheld or withdrawn in certain circumstances, though it is not permissible to forgo ordinary treatment. Extraordinary treatment has been perceived as the use of high technology, such as respirators and invasive measures. Despite the attempts to give precision to these terms, they are confusing and not helpful medically or ethically. It is best to avoid such language when considering treatment options or presenting the treatment options to the competent patient or surrogate decision-maker. *Treatment can be either ordinary or extraordinary depending on the particular use of the treatment.*[11]

The more relevant considerations are 1) the resulting balance between the benefits and the burdens (or harms) of treatment in relationship to the overall management goals of the patient and 2) to treat according to the patient's assessment or the surrogate's understanding of the patient's desires. When the patient or surrogate decides that the burdens of treatment are greater than the benefits to be accrued, the house officer is not obligated to begin or continue the treatment. If the patient decides to begin treatment, but after a period of time the benefits are not achieved, the physician should review the decision with the patient in light of the more accurate facts. The labeling of treatments as ordinary or extraordinary is not only misleading but can lead to confusion.

Active and Passive Euthanasia

Much of the literature on the subject of euthanasia tries to distinguish between active and passive euthanasia by pointing out the difference between acts of omission and commission or the ordinary and extraordinary distinction or hastening death and killing. Several court rulings have attempted to apply these distinctions.[12,13] However, the frequently discussed differences do not seem very satisfactory when applied in the clinical setting. A more helpful way of distinguishing between the two emotionally laden concepts is presented by Culver and Gert.[4] They indicate that a competent patient's valid refusal of treatment determines what is to be done or not done, even when the action or refraining from the action will result in the patient's death. When the house officer accepts the terminal cancer patient's refusal of life-sustaining treatment, such as writing a Do Not Resuscitate order, not starting antibiotics, or removing the respirator, the physician is performing passive, voluntary (patient has consented) euthanasia that is morally justified. *Passive euthanasia is the same as a valid refusal of treatment that will hasten the patient's death.* In such situations, it is best not to even use the term euthanasia because of the confusion and misunderstandings about the word.

What if the terminally ill cancer patient requests that the physician give him an injection of medication to directly kill him? This would be called active euthanasia. Some argue that active euthanasia, the direct killing of the patient, would be a merciful act.[14] Despite the altruistic goals, the issue may be the result of an incorrect premise, in that the patient should not have to suffer from pain. "Modern methods of pain management enable physicians and nurses to control pain in virtually all such patients without the use of lethal poisons, though sometimes at the cost of so sedating the patient that interaction and communication with others is limited or no longer possible."[15] Besides the issue of increasing the physician's skills in pain control there is no moral requirement for house officers to abide by a patient's request for such actions in comparison to the moral significance of the patient making valid refusal of treatment.[16] This line of reasoning is similar to the physician not being obligated to perform abortions or penile implants even though the patient makes such a request.

There is also reasonable concern about potential abuse by physicians in performing active euthanasia. Elderly cancer patients who are an emotional and financial burden to their families may be vulnerable to having their lives wrongly ended.[15] House officers and other physicians may find their role as a health care provider undermined by their willingness to actively kill patients. This could also have a dramatic impact on society's view of the physician.

INTENDED AND UNINTENDED CONSQUENCES OF MEDICATIONS

I have argued that the *intentional, direct ending of a human life is morally wrong while allowing a patient to die is morally justified*. How is this understanding applied to the issue of administering medication to the terminally ill patient in severe pain? This problem concerns the important distinction between intended and unintended consequences. The distinction is a component of the Roman Catholic Doctrine of Double Effect.[9] In the situation of a patient in extreme pain due to bone metastases, a house officer may consider increasing the amount of morphine to control the pain but at the same time may be concerned about depressing the respirations to the point of hastening the death. Assuming the house officer has obtained the consent from the patient or surrogate after discussing the potential risks, benefits, and alternatives of the medication, it is morally appropriate to administer the medication because the intention is to relieve the patient's suffering. If the intention is to kill, it is not morally justified. One should not gain pain relief through an act intended to kill. On the other hand, if the purpose is the relief of pain and the patient consents, accepting the risks, including the hastening of death, there is moral justification.

DECISION-MAKING DISAGREEMENTS

In an ideal world, patients, families, and physicians would always agree on the ethically correct treatment decisions, but in the house officer's world, disagreements are common. Despite this fact, *most disagreements can be ironed out by discussion, reason, and compromise.* Cancer patients may ethically refuse treatments. Physicians may personally disagree with the decision but should respect the competent patient's rational refusal. Physicians, on the other hand, have no obligation to perform treatments they find medically or ethically objectionable on any patient.

Another potential disagreement involves the terminally ill patient who wants "everything possible done" and the physician who believes such a decision is inappropriate. A common example is the patient who insists upon full resuscitation when dying of widespread metastatic cancer despite the counsel of the physician that this effort cannot possibly help the patient. This difficult situation usually indicates poor communication. Some patients fear that if they agree to DNR status, the physician will abandon them to suffer a slow, painful death. Honest communication concerning the harm of CPR, the poor outcome results, and the reassurance that general comfort support will be provided can promote a reasoned decision. If, however, the patient is adamant about their desire for CPR, the house officer should honor the request. The discussion should include a clarification of whether the patient would want life support if a "successful" resuscitation would leave the patient in a coma. One way of avoiding disagreements is to not offer futile treatments.

Occasionally, disagreements occur within the medical team or between the house officer and the nursing staff. Such situations should not be ignored and should be dealt with openly through honest and direct communication. Frequently, these disagreements are caused by misunderstandings over the facts of the case or treatment options. *Many ethical dilemmas are really disagreements over the facts of the health status and desires of the cancer patient or the management goals, and the potential benefits of treatments.* Improved communication can decrease most of these conflicts. Regular team meetings with all members of the health care team can reduce such conflicts. House officers may consider inviting nurses, chaplains, and social workers to participate on morning rounds or team meetings.

Disagreements occur within families having to make decisions for an incompetent patient. This may be the result of "hidden agendas," such as guilt or anger toward the patient. If a family member has not been designated the decision-maker a family consensus is essential. Such families should receive appropriate counseling, and non-emergency treatment decisions should be suspended until consensus is achieved.[5]

ETHICS ADVISORY COMMITTEES

House officers may want to discuss an ethical dilemma with a multidisciplinary committee made up of professionals with knowledge in clinical ethics. *Many hospitals have established Ethics Advisory Committees (EAC) in response to the growing number of ethical issues in health care and the recognition that many health care providers feel uncertain in the midst of such situations.* The purpose of an EAC varies to some extent at each hospital but in general serves as a forum for health care providers to discuss ethical issues that relate to patient care with professionals capable of applying ethical theories and concepts to the ethical issues. Although there has been some skepticism expressed by physicians about the need for EAC, these committees have continued to grow in numbers and, where they are functioning well, serve as a valuable resource to house officers and other health care professionals. A 1985 survey indicated that 60 percent of hospitals with more than 200 beds had functioning committees.[17] There is no doubt that this figure is much higher today.

The composition of an EAC's may include physicians, nurses, chaplains, administrators, legal counsel, social workers, and ethicists. The criteria for membership is motivation, time, and a willingness to develop knowledge about clinical ethics.

There are three basic functions of the EAC. The first is an educational role. The EAC facilitates various activities to increase the understanding of hospital personnel of how to employ ethical reasoning to ethical dilemmas. House officers should consider inviting the chair of the EAC to lead a regular "Ethics Case Conference" or participate in other educational forums. The second role is one of policy review and drafting. The EAC is frequently involved in recommending hospital policy concerning such topics as "Limitation of Therapy," "AIDS Testing," and "Terminal Care Documents." The third role, case consultation, is most relevant to house officers.[18,19] *When a house officer is uncertain about an ethical dilemma, he or she can contact the chair of the EAC for advice.* The EAC usually has several members of the committee review the particular case, applying systematic ethical reasoning. The case is then discussed with the medical team. *The advice is intended to help the physician in the natural decision process between the patient and care provider and not to dictate any management plan.* It is a similar process to other consultants providing professional advice which the primary physician must decide to use.

GENERAL CLINICAL GUIDELINES

The care of cancer patients occurs within the framework of three basic factors: (1) the characteristics of the disease process, (2) the characteristics of the patient and family, and (3) the characteristics of the house officer. How these factors relate influences the quality of care and occasionally the quality of death.[20]

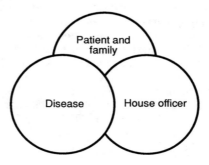

Inherent in this interrelationship is the potential for ethical dilemmas. How the house officer responds to these dilemmas directly impacts on the patient's care and the physician's growth during the training years. Essential to the ethical care of cancer patients is open and honest communication concerning the diagnosis and prognosis. *The patient must be made fully aware of his or her situation.* From this foundation a trusting physician/patient relationship is formed. The patient then can be offered treatment options and is free to accept or refuse such treatments. During these conversations, the house officer should insure that emotional support for the patient is fostered through the medical team or by resources such as the chaplain, psychiatrist, or social worker. *House officers should be able to anticipate problems and should discuss them with the patient, such as resuscitation status.* Since many ethical issues involve incompetent patients, the best way to deal with ethical problems is to anticipate them and discuss them openly with the patient before they become incompetent including identifying the proxy decision-makers. *Talking about ethical issues may seem like another burden for the overworked, stressed, and tired house officer, yet in the long run, dealing with the dilemmas prior to their occurence can reduce time consuming and frustrating problems.* When ethical problems occur, the house officer should apply systematic reasoning and should not be reluctant to use the available resources, such as the hospital Ethics Advisory Committee.

REFERENCES

1. American College of Physicians Ethics Manual: Part 1: history; the patient; other physicians. *Ann Intern Med* 111 N(3):245–252, 1989.
2. Gert, B: *Morality: A New Justification of the Moral Rules.* Oxford, England, Oxford University Press, 1988.
3. Gert, B, Nelson, W.A., Culver, C.: Moral theory and neurology. *Neurol Clin* 7:681–696, 1989.
4. Culver, C.M., Gert, B.: Ethical issues in oncology. *Psych Med* 5 (4):389–404, 1987.
5. Nelson, W.A., Bernat, J.L.: Decisions to withhold and terminate treatment. *Neurol Clin* 7:759–774, 1989.
6. Emanuel, L.L., Emanuel, E.J.: The medical directive. *JAMA* 261(22):3288–3293, 1989.
7. Lo, B., et al: Patient attitudes to discussing life-sustaining treatment. *Arch Intern Med* 146:1614, 1986.
8. Ruark, J.E., Ruffin, T.A., et al: Initiating and withdrawing life support: principles and practice in adult medicine. *N Engl J Med* 318(25):26, 1988.
9. Jonsen, A.R., et al: *Clinical Ethics.* New York, MacMillian Publishing Company, 1986.
10. Jennings,B., et al: Ethical challenges of chronic illness. Hastings Center Report 18 (1):1, 1988.
11. Wanzer, S.H., Federman, M.D., Adelstein, S.J., et al: The physician's responsibility toward hopelessly ill patients. *N Engl J Med* 320 (13):844–849, 1989.
12. Barber and Nedil v. Superior Court. 195 Cal Rptr. 484 (Cal. App. 2 Dist.), 1983.
13. In re Conroy. 486 A.2d 1209 (N.J. 1985).
14. Rachels, J.: Active and passive euthanasia. *N Engl J Med:* 292:78, 1975.
15. Brock, D.: Death and dying. In Veatch, R.M. (ed): *Medical Ethics.* Boston, Jones and Bartlett Publishers, 1989, p. 348.
16. Culver, C.M., Gert, B.: Distinguishing between active and passive euthanasia. *Geratrics Clinics* 2:1,1986.
17. Ethics committees double since '83: survey. *Hospitals,* 59(21):60–61, 1985.
18. Perkins, H.S., Saathoff, B.S.: Impact of medical ethics consultations on physicians: an exploratory study. *Am J Med* 85:761–764, 1988.
19. Siegler, M., Singer, M.D.: Clinical ethics consultations: godsend or "god squad?" *Am J Med* 85:759–760, 1988.
20. Mogielnicki, R.P., Nelson, W., Dulac, J., Quality of death study of hospitalized veterans. *J Can Ed* 5 (2):135–145, 1990.

Chapter 14

Selected Procedures in Medical Oncology

VENOUS ACCESS

The ability to gain reliable venous access has become a major element in the care of cancer patients. While oncology nurse specialists have assumed the major responsibility for the administration of chemotherapeutic agents, all physicians and health care professionals involved in the care of cancer patients should have a fundamental understanding of the various venous access devices available and the common complications seen with use of these devices.

Not all patients undergoing chemotherapy require central venous access. If a patient is to receive simple monthly intravenous bolus injections of chemotherapy for a defined period of time, central venous access is usually not required. Because of the risk of infection and other complications, a central venous access device should not be placed simply for blood drawing or the convenience of the staff. Table 14.1 lists the indications for central venous access.

A number of permanent central venous access devices have been developed. These fall into two broad categories: 1) percutaneous silicone silastic atrial catheters (Hickman-Broviac), and 2) implantable ports (Mediport, Port-A-Cath). Permanent percutaneous intravenous catheters were first introduced to administer parenteral hyperalimentation (Broviac). These were later used for the administration of chemotherapy (Hickman). Today, double and triple lumen catheters allow the simultaneous administration of chemotherapy, intravenous antibiotics, and blood products as well as blood drawing.

Table 14.1
Indications for Central Venous Access

---

a. Limited peripheral access
b. Frequent venous access required
c. Continuous infusion of chemotherapy (especially vesicants)
d. Total parenteral nutrition (TPN)
e. Frequent administration of blood products
f. Bone marrow transplantation
g. Acute leukemia, high grade lymphoma
h. Home infusion therapy

Percutaneous silicone silastic atrial catheters (Hickman-Broviac) are surgically inserted into the subclavian vein by tunneling the catheter subcutaneously through the skin of the chest wall into the subclavian vein with the tip resting in the superior vena cava or right atrium. These are then securely fastened to the skin of the chest and can remain in place for years if necessary. Since these catheters violate the skin barrier there is an increased risk of infection through direct access of bacteria. Strict adherence to sterile technique when changing catheter dressings and accessing the catheter ports can avoid this complication. There also may be a restriction in lifestyle and occupation that is caused by having a catheter protruding through the skin. However, this is offset by the ready access gained to the ports on these devices and the availability of multiple ports (Table 14.2).

More recently a number of implantable subcutaneous catheters have been developed (Mediport, Port A Cath). These devices consist of a self-sealing silicone septum as an access port, a metal hub, and a radio-opaque catheter. The port and hub portion of these devices are inserted into a pocket created under the skin, usually in the subclavian area on the chest wall. The catheter portion is inserted into the subclavian vein and superior vena cava. These have the benefit of being totally subcutaneous and thus have the theoretic advantage of a lower rate of infection, less maintenance, and greater patient acceptability. Access into these catheters is more difficult and requires a special needle called a Huber needle. Table 14.2 contrasts the various indications for the insertions of the two major types of permanent central venous access devices.

Table 14.2

Implantable vs. Percutaneous Venous Access Devices

Implantable Ports (Mediport, Port A Cath)	Percutaneous (Hickman-Broviac)
—Intermittent infrequent access required	—Frequent venous access required
—Intermittent bolus injections of chemotherapy (non-vesicant)	—Simultaneous administration of multiple medications
—Long term out-patient chemotherapy	—Continuous infusion of chemotherapy
—Infrequent blood sampling	—Frequent use of blood products
—Patient occupation or lifestyle	—Frequent blood sampling
	—Total parenteral nutrition
	—Bone marrow transplantation
	—Acute leukemia

Many different types of temporary central venous access devices have also been developed. These are primarily used in the intensive care setting or when emergency venous access is required. These may on occasion be indicated for the short term administration of chemotherapy, antibiotics, TPN, or hydration.

When accessing any central venous catheter a clamp should always be readily available because of the danger of air embolism. When not in use all tubing should be clamped, and an open port should never be left unattended. As little as 70–100cc of air can be fatal.

Method of drawing blood from Hickman type catheter:

1. Wear gloves.
2. Swab red cap of Hickman with alcohol swab. The red lumen is the largest lumen.
3. Cautiously pierce the cap of the tubing, being extremely careful not to puncture the tubing. Alternatively, the cap may be unscrewed and a threaded syringe attached.
4. Unclamp Hickman.
5. With a 6cc syringe draw up 4cc of blood for discard, then reclamp.
6. Pierce cap or, if you have removed cap, screw onto the Hickman a large enough syringe to obtain blood specimen.

7. Unclamp, obtain specimen, reclamp.
8. When specimens obtained, remove syringe and attach another syringe with 5cc normal saline to Hickman, unclamp, flush and reclamp when flushing the last 0.5cc.
9. If cap was removed to draw blood, prime new Hickman cap with heparin (1cc of 25U/cc); remove normal saline syringe from Hickman, screw on new cap.
10. Flush line with either 2.5cc of 25U/cc. heparin flush or 5cc of 10U/cc flush, reclamping Hickman when flushing the last 0.5cc.
11. If the cap was not removed, the above flushing can be accomplished by piercing the cap with needle on syringe.

Method for accessing implantable ports:

1. The overlying skin over the diaphram of the catheter is prepared with Betadine solution (3×) and wiped with alcohol.
2. Using sterile gloves the hub of the diaphram of the catheter is grasped between the thumb and forefinger and the Huber needle is inserted perpendicular to the port septum.
3. Location is verified by aspiration of blood to confirm the location of the tip of the Huber needle within the reservoir of the hub.
4. Blood drawing or infusion therapy can be performed when the location of the Huber needle is confirmed.
5. When the procedure is complete the hub and tubing is flushed with 20cc of sterile saline.
6. The system is flushed with 5cc of heparin (25U/cc).

COMPLICATIONS

Infection

Infection is one of the most common and serious complications of parenteral therapy. Infection rates as high as 19% have been reported with central venous catheters. The rate of infectious complication can be reduced if strict sterile technique is observed. This becomes especially important in the immunosuppressed and neutropenic host.

Infection caused by intravenous catheters can be divided into two broad categories: 1) local insertion site and 2) systemic sepsis. Local infection usually occurs when there is a break in sterile technique or a peripheral venous catheter is left in place longer than 72 hours. Studies have shown that the rate of infection rises with the duration that the peripheral catheter remains in place, and it is now virtually a universal nursing policy to change all peripheral catheters every 72 hours. The number of infections increases with the number of ports on a central venous access device. Therefore, the number of ports should be kept to the minimum required when selecting a device. One port should be dedicated to TPN alone if this is anticipated, and this port should not be violated except for TPN.

Local infectious complications include insertion site infection, tunnel tract or pocket infection, and septic thrombophlebitis. Insertion site infections are local infections of the tissue at the point where the catheter exits the skin and they present with local pain and erythema at the catheter insertion site. Occasionally a purulent exudate is present. If these signs are present in a peripheral site the catheter should be removed immediately. Patients with central venous access devices should be placed on 10 days of oral antibiotic therapy to cover the most commonly encountered organisms (usually oral dicloxacillin, 250mg. PO QID). In the febrile neutropenic host, intravenous antibiotics must be started, since this represents a possible source of fever and sepsis (usually vancomycin 1g. IV q8h). Insertion site infection can usually be treated without catheter removal.

Tunnel infections are local infections of the subcutaneous tissue around the tubing track that extends proximally from the skin exit wound and along the tubing to the site of entry into the central vein. Pocket infections are infections of the subcutaneous tissue around the metal hub of an implantable port. Both are characterized by pain and erythema over the catheter tubing (or hub) where it travels in the subcutaneous tissues of the chest wall. This usually indicates that the tract of the catheter tubing (or hub) is colonized with bacteria. Both of these types of catheter related infection require catheter removal. Studies have shown that in 60–80% of cases, these infections cannot be cleared even with intravenous antibiotics. Because the catheter acts as a foreign body, it often cannot be sterilized and represents a source of recurrent infection.

All neutropenic patients with local infections and all patients with tunnel tract or pocket infections should receive intravenous antibiotics. In non-neutropenic patients, insertion site infections can be treated with oral antibiotics and local care alone, with intravenous antibiotics reserved for nonresponders. If the infection progresses or the patient deteriorates even with IV antibiotics, the catheter should be removed. In neutropenic patients with tunnel tract or pocket infections, a short course of IV antibiotics can be attempted with rapid removal of the catheter if the patient is non-responsive. In general, catheter removal must depend on the individual circumstances.

One of the most serious 'local' infectious complications is the development of septic thrombophlebitis. This occurs most commonly in patients receiving TPN either peripherally or through a central access device. In this case, the actual lumen of the vein and associated clot become infected and continuously seed microorganisms into the blood stream. This is characterized by overwhelming and refractory sepsis and requires removal of the catheter and (frequently) surgical excision of the involved vessel.

The clinical features of catheter related sepsis are indistinguishable from bacteremia arising from other sites. If a patient with a central catheter develops a fever without an obvious source of infection, catheter related sepsis must always be considered. In both the neutropenic and non-neutropenic patient, blood cultures should be obtained from both a peripheral site and from the catheter port(s) (all ports must be cultured with 2–3 lumen catheters).

Sepsis or bacteremia due to catheter related infection is diagnosed when blood cultures are positive from both the catheter lumen and/or a peripheral site (Table 14.3). Using semiquantitative cultures the colony count from the catheter specimen should be higher than the peripheral specimen. A high index of suspicion is needed because the cultures are frequently negative.

The most commonly isolated organisms are Gram positive, coagulase negative staphylococci (*S. epidermidis*). This is followed closely by coagulase positive *S. aureus*. The other common organisms isolated are listed in Table 14.4. Fungal infections are unusual except in patients on TPN. Isolation of S. epidermidis or diptheroids cannot be ignored as a 'skin contaminant,' especially in the septic neutropenic patient, and must be acted upon until an alternative source of infection is documented.

In the past, infection of a venous access device usually dictated removal to assure eradication of the infection. However, a number of recent studies have demonstrated that catheter removal is not always necessary.

Table 14.3
Findings in Catheter Related Sepsis

1. Catheter culture positive and peripheral culture positive for the same organism.
2. Catheter culture positive for the same organism on 2 occasions.
3. Catheter culture positive and skin insertion site positive for the same organism.
4. Catheter culture positive and peripheral cultures negative in the absence of other sources of infection.
5. Peripheral culture positive without obvious other sources of infection (*Staphylococcus epidermidis, Staphylococcus aureus*)
6. Tenderness and induration at insertion site or over subcutaneous tubing (tunnel tract or pocket infection).

Table 14.4
Common Organisms in Central Venous Catheter Infection

Organism	Percentage
Gram Positives	60–70%
—*S. epidermidis*	
—*S. aureus*	
—*Streptococci (Viridans* and *Grp. D)*	
—*Corynebacterium* spp.	
—*J K Diptheroid* spp.	
Gram Negatives	20–30%
—*Escherichia coli*	
—*Bacillus* spp.	
—*Acinetobacter* spp.	
—*Pseudomonas aeruginosa, cepacia*	
—*Enterobacter* spp.	
—*Citrobacter* spp.	
—*Escherichia coli*	
—*Serratia marcescens*	
—*Klebsiella pneumoniae*	
Yeast/Fungi	5–10%
—*Candida albicans, tropicalis*	
—*Aspergillus* spp.	

Empiric antibiotic coverage should be started early; usually an amino-glycoside and vancomycin are administered. If a temporary central venous catheter is in place, the catheter should be replaced over a wire and the tip cultured. If the catheter tip culture is positive the catheter must be removed (colonized insertion site) and a new one reinserted at an alternative site.

With permanent percutaneous or subcutaneous devices, recent data have shown that more than 80% of infections with coagulase negative staphylococci can be cleared by treating directly through the catheter with a 10 day course of intravenous vancomycin. All ports must be treated. If cultures are positive after 48–72 hours despite appropriate antibiotic treatment, the catheter must be removed. The indications for catheter removal are given in Table 14.5. In patients with persistently positive blood cultures an echocardiogram should be performed to rule out endocarditis.

Extravasation

One of the most debilitating complications of the administration of chemotherapeutic agents is extravasation into the subcutaneous tissues of vesicant cytotoxic agents. The most common vesicants are listed in Table 14.6. Irritants do not cause permanent damage but may cause pain and inflammation at the catheter site and vein. All vesicant chemotherapy should be administered through a central line whenever possible. A peripheral intravenous catheter must be tested with intravenous fluids first at a high flow rate to determine the patency of the vessel to be used and to exclude extravasation prior to the administration of chemotherapy. Never use the dorsum of the hand or volar aspect of the wrist. If there

Table 14.5
Indications for Central Venous Access Device Removal

1. Documented catheter related infection not responsive to appropriate antibiotic therapy; (24 hr neutropenic, 72 hr non-neutropenic).
2. Tunnel tract or pocket infection.
3. *Candida* or *Bacillus* spp. isolated.
4. Relapse of infection after appropriate course of antibiotics.
5. Catheter tip culture positive (temporary catheters).

Table 14.6
Vesicant and Irritant Chemotherapeutic Agents

Vesicant	Irritant
Vincristine	Etoposide (VP16)
Vinblastine	Tenoposide (VM26)
Daunorubicin	Streptozocin
Doxorubicin	Carmustine (BCNU)
Dactinomycin	Cisplatin
Mithramycin	Dacarbazine (DTIC)
Mitomycin	
Nitrogen mustard	

is any doubt about the patency of the vessel, the infusion should not be attempted. There are almost no circumstances in oncology in which the administration of a chemotherapeutic agent cannot be delayed several days if necessary to obtain adequate intravenous access.

Extravasation usually causes immediate, intense pain but may on occasion be painless. The pain is usually followed by erythema and edema within a few hours and increasing induration within a few days. Skin ulceration and skin necrosis can occur within 1–3 weeks and may lead to necrosis of the underlying fascia, tendon, and periosteum. If this is not recognized early, surgical intervention and wide local excision and debridement is necessary. If this occurs on the dorsum of the hand or volar aspect of the wrist, severe permanent disability can result and even require amputation of the involved extremity.

If there is any question of a possible extravasation the infusion should be stopped immediately. The most effective treatment of extravasation is controversial. No large randomized studies exist and most of the data are based on animal models. Some clinicians recommend only conservative management with elevation of the involved extremity and ice compresses or heat as indicated. Others recommend specific intervention based on the type of agent extravasated. General measures in the treatment of extravasation are discussed in Table 14.7.

The concept behind the administration of most antidotes is to disperse the chemotherapy and to facilitate its absorption from the subcutaneous tissues. Reference material or the package insert should be consulted

Table 14.7
General Measures

1. Stop the infusion
2. Attempt to draw any remaining chemotherapy out of the tubing and needle hub, and leave the needle in place (optional).
3. Inject the antidote through the needle and in a clockwise order subcutaneously around the site of extravasation (optional). A 25 gage needle should be used and changed with each injection.
4. Apply light dressings.
5. Elevate the arm.
6. Apply ice packs if indicated.
7. Photograph and arrange early (plastic) surgical evaluation.

whenever an extravasation occurs because the type of specific intervention depends on the agent extravasated. The treatment of some of the most common vesicants are discussed below.

Antidote Recommendations

Plant alkyloids—vincristine, vinblastine, VP 16. Inject 1–6 ml of hyaluronidase (Wydase 150U/ml) into the subcutaneous tissue around the site of extravasation in a clockwise manner. The subcutaneous dosing should be repeated several times over the next 3–4 hours. Warm compresses should then be applied to the area to aid absorption. Hyaluronidase may enhance absorption and dispersion of the extravasated drug. Corticosteroids and cooling appear to worsen toxicity.

Anthracycline antibiotics—doxorubicin (Adriamycin), daunomycin (Cerubidine). Cold compresses may inhibit the cytotoxicity of the drug. Local injection of low dose corticosteroids may be helpful; hydrocortisone (100 mg/ml) 0.5–1.0 ml solution intravenously or subcutaneously; dexamethasone 0.5–1.0 ml of 4 mg/ml solution IV or SC. If pain, erythema, and/or swelling persist beyond 48 hours, debridement may be necessary and the patient should be referred immediately to a plastic surgeon.

Alkylating agents—mechlorethiamine (nitrogen mustard). Isotonic sodium thiosulfate (1 gm/10ml) (4 ml of 10% sodium thiosulfate with 6 ml sterile water = 1/6 molar solution) is injected through the existing IV line and SC into the site of extravasation. Repeated subcutaneous dosing should be performed several times over the next 3–4 hours. Cold compresses should be applied and treatment should be initiated immediately.

Mitomycin C (Mutamycin)—Cold compresses should be applied. Topical DMSO should be applied over the area of extravasation: 1–2 ml of 1M mol DMSO 50–100%. Use of DMSO is considered investigational.

For other agents, the specific manufacturer's recommendations should be followed. Remember, the best way to prevent extravasation is to secure adequate (central) venous access before an infusion is started.

Clotting

Obstruction of the catheter is a commonly encountered problem. Usually this is the result of a clot at the catheter tip or obstruction by the right atrial wall. If unable to draw blood from the line, it should be gently flushed with 3 ml (percutaneous) or 6 ml (subcutaneous) of 1:1000 heparin. The pressure should not be excessive because the catheter tubing can rupture if enough pressure is exerted. If flushing fails, 3 ml. of urokinase 5000IU (Abbokinase) may be instilled into the tubing and hub. After 5 minutes aspiration should be attempted again. If this fails this procedure can be repeated using a 30 min incubation time until the clot is dissolved. No more than 3 doses should be given.

Venous thrombosis is a relatively uncommon complication with central devices. Symptoms include aching discomfort or acute pain in the shoulder, neck, or arm on the same side as the catheter insertion site. Later supraclavicular, ipsilateral arm and neck swelling and venous dilatation similar to superior vena cava syndrome may develop. If central venous thrombosis is suspected, vesicant chemotherapy should never be infused through the catheter because severe phlebitis and extravasation may result. The patient should have a chest x-ray to confirm the position of the catheter tip, followed by a venogram done though an ipsilateral peripheral vein.

If a central venous thrombosis is documented the central venous access device must be removed. Frequently the patency of the vessel can be reestablished with the use of streptokinase or tissue plasminogen activator if administered rapidly after the symptoms develop. Streptokinase is administered at a slow rate through an ipsilateral vein or systemically.

When patency is reestablished, systemic anticoagulation is undertaken with heparin, and when indicated, coumadin.

Hickman/Mediport declotting procedures:

1. Once inability to draw blood through venous access device has been determined, access line and flush with normal saline (3cc Hickman, 6cc Mediport) to remove the heparin from the tubing.
2. The urokinase dose equals the catheter volume (3cc Hickman, 6cc Mediport). Note: Urokinase concentration is 5000U/ml.
3. Attach the syringe containing the urokinase, unclamp the catheter and slowly instill the urokinase. Reclamp the catheter.
4. Leave the urokinase in catheter for 5 minutes. Then unclamp catheter and aspirate with syringe. If you are unable to aspirate blood, clamp the catheter and wait another 5 minutes after instilling the urokinase. Repeat this procedure, then wait 30 minutes and attempt aspiration again. If unable to draw blood after one hour, remove the syringe and place another (fresh) dose of dose of urokinase into the tubing. This may be repeated three times.
5. Following successful aspiration the Hickman or Mediport should be flushed as described above.

Intrathecal Drug Administration

The presentation of carcinomatous meningitis (CM) is discussed in chapter 15. Both radiation therapy and chemotherapy are used to treat CM. This usually consists of low dose radiation therapy (2500–3000 Rad to either the entire neuroaxis—i.e. the whole brain and spinal cord—or to specific sites of involvement). Radiation therapy may be given concurrently with intrathecal chemotherapy. Intrathecal chemotherapy can be administered via lumbar puncture or via an implantable Omaya intraventricular reservoir. If the patient has reasonable life expectancy and frequent repetitive intrathecal drug administration is anticipated, an Omaya reservoir should be inserted.

Three medications are widely used for intrathecal therapy in clinical oncology. These are methotrexate, thiotepa, and cytosine arabinoside (Table 14.8). These can be administered either through lumbar puncture or through an implantable Omaya reservoir. When a lumbar puncture or an Omaya reservoir is used, an isovolumetric amount of CSF is removed

Table 14.8
Intrathecal Medications

Methotrexate*
10–15 mg twice weekly until CSF clears, then monthly. Folinic acid rescue may be necessary if the patient is receiving concurrent systemic chemotherapy (10 mg PO every 6 h for 8 doses to begin 24 h after initial dose of methotrexate).
Side effects—headache, arachnoiditis, leukoencephalopathy, myelopathy, motor dysfunction, depression, leukopenia, mucositis.
Thiotepa*
10 mg twice weekly until CSF clears, then monthly.
Side effects—headache, myelopathy, motor dysfunction, variable cognitive dysfunction.
Cytosine arabinoside*
30–100 mg/m^2 twice weekly until CSF clears.
Side effects—headache, nausea, vomiting, fever, arachnoiditis, encephalomyelopathy, seizures, cerebellar degeneration, paralysis.

---

*All drugs must be resuspended in preservative-free, isotonic, non-bacteriostatic solution only.

and an equal volume of drug in a preservative free diluent is injected slowly (Table 14.9). The patient should remain supine for several hours to allow equal dispersion of the drug. Therapy is usually continued on a twice weekly basis until the CSF clears.

Methotrexate is the most studied and most frequently used agent. No advantage to combination therapy has been demonstrated. Thiotepa and cytosine arabinoside are generally employed in patients resistant to methotrexate. One can expect response rates between 40–79%, but even with therapy, survival is poor.

THORACENTESIS-PLEURTHORACENTESIS-PLEURODESIS

Indications

Pleural effusions are frequently encountered in cancer patients. However, not all effusions are malignant in origin, and it is important to determine the exact nature of the effusion prior to starting specific therapy.

Table 14.9

Accessing an Omaya Intraventricular Reservoir

---

1. Patient should be supine.
2. The rubber port of the reservoir should be located under the scalp by palpation.
3. Shave area of hair (with safety razor) if growth is heavy.
4. Wipe area over port with Betadine swab (3X).
5. Wear sterile gloves.
6. Cleanse port with sterile alcohol swab (3X).
7. Attach a 10cc syringe to 23 g butterfly needle.
8. Puncture the skin perpendicular to the septum.
9. Gently draw off CSF specimen. Draw off an amount equal to the amount of drug and diluent to be injected.
10. Pinch off tubing, disconnect syringe with CSF and attach syringe with intrathecal chemotherapy.
11. Inject chemotherapy slowly over 5–10 minutes. Do not inject air.
12. Pinch off tubing again and attach 3 cc syringe with lactated Ringer's solution. Instill just enough into the port to clear the tubing of chemotherapy (1–3 cc).
13. Remove butterfly needle and apply pressure until bleeding stops.

Malignant pleural effusions can develop through a number of mechanisms. Lymphatic obstruction either by tumor involvement of the mediastinal lymph nodes or lymphangitic spread can lead to diminished lymphatic drainage from the pleural surface and a chylous effusion. Direct tumor involvement of the visceral or parietal pleura is the most common mechanism and usually leads to bloody, exudative effusions.

The most common malignant tumors causing pleural effusions are: lung carcinoma, breast carcinoma, ovarian carcinoma, gastric carcinoma, lymphoma, and melanoma. The rate of development and prognosis depends on the biology of the particular neoplasm. Overall, the prognosis for patients with malignant effusion is quite poor with a median survival of only 3–6 months.

The most common presenting symptoms of a malignant pleural effusion are cough, dyspnea, and (pleuritic) chest pain. However, about 25% will be asymptomatic at presentation. Decreased breath sounds, dullness to percussion, decreased fremitus and undetectable diaphramatic excursion are the most common physical findings. In extreme cases, the patient may be tachypneic with tracheal deviation to the contralateral side of the effusion.

PA and lateral chest x-rays should be obtained along with lateral decubitus views. Characteristically, there is blunting of the costophrenic angle with a variable degree of opacification. There may or may not be layering of the fluid, depending on whether loculation is present.

A diagnostic thoracentesis should be performed in all patients suspected of having a malignant effusion (Table 14.10). Characteristically, these will be exudative in nature with an elevated protein and LDH but on occasion may be transudative. The fluid is usually serosanguinous. In approximately 50% of the cases the cytologic analysis will be negative. There is usually a moderate leukocytosis. CEA levels when elevated are highly suggestive of malignancy.

The management of malignant pleural effusions involves drainage of the fluid with either simple thoracentesis or chest tube drainage and pleural sclerotherapy (pleurodesis). Simple thoracentesis can produce rapid relief of symptoms but the effusion recurs in over 90% of patients unless a pleurodesis procedure is performed. However, simple thoracentesis will allow analysis of the pleural fluid and give important characteristics such as whether the fluid can be drained (loculation present) and if chest tube drainage is indicated. It will also allow determination of the rate of reaccumulation.

Before pleurodesis is performed, one should determine whether the cause of the effusion is central lymphatic obstruction or direct involvement of plerual surface by tumor. In general, effusions due to central

Table 14.10
Malignant Pleural Fluid Characteristics

Exudative
—Protein > 3 grams/dl or pleural to serum ratio > 0.5
—LDH > 225 IU or pleural to serum ratio > 0.6
—WBC > 2500
—pH > 7.2
—Elevated CEA (90% specificity)
—Cytology positive in 50%

---

lymphatic obstruction do not respond to pleurodesis. A pleurodesis should not be performed in a patient with a limited life expectancy. If the patient is asymptomatic and there is only a slow rate of accumulation, a pleurodesis is not indicated. The major indication for pleurodesis occurs in a patient with a symptomatic malignant effusion which resolves with simple thoracentesis, which rapidly reaccumulates. The life expectancy should be greater than 3 months.

Technique

A number of agents have been advocated for pleurodesis. Tetracycline has gained the widest use because of its effectiveness, low cost, and low morbidity. It is effective in approximately 60–80% of cases when properly administered. A number of chemotherapeutic agents have also been used including bleomycin, thiotepa, fluorouracil, and nitrogen mustard, but none of these are convincingly superior to tetracycline. These agents are not used for their antineoplastic properties but rather the intense pleural reaction they cause. They can be absorbed from the pleural space causing nausea, vomiting, and bone marrow suppression. Other agents including talcum powder, radioactive isotopes, and quinacrine (antimalarial) have also been used. A surgical pleurectomy is rarely if ever indicated.

Prior to pleural sclerotherapy a chest tube must be inserted. This procedure is preferably performed by an experienced surgeon to minimize the pain and discomfort of the procedure. The tube is inserted in the most dependent portion of the lung. The pleural fluid is allowed to drain by gravity and later by suction set to water seal. All the fluid must be drained before pleurodesis is attempted. Because the injection of the tetracycline or other sclerosing agent produces an intense pleuritis that can be painful, the patient should be given either systemic analgesia or local anesthesia into the pleural space with lidocaine hydrochloride. With the proper selection of patients and proper technique, malignant effusions can be controlled in 80–90% of patients (Table 14.11). Most failures are due to injecting the sclerosing agents into patients whose plerual space is not completely drained by the chest tube or who have a central lymphatic obstruction. The key to success of the procedure is the intense pleuritis produced by the tetracycline (or other agent) and the approximation of the visceral and parietal pleura by the chest tube so that a pleural scarring and syndesis can occur.

Table 14.11
Intrapleural Injection of Sclerosing Agent

---

1. Underlying lung re-expanded.
2. Lidocaine 150 mg in 50 cc NS should be slowly injected directly through the chest tube.
3. Over the next 10–15 minutes the patient is repositioned frequently to allow dispersion of the anesthetic.
4. Tetracycline 14 mg/kg diluted to total volume of 50 ml is injected slowly through the chest tube. An additional 50cc of saline is injected through the tubing to clear the tetracycline.
5. The chest tubed is clamped.
6. The patient is repositioned frequently over the next 2 hours.
7. The chest tube is unclamped and attached to suction for at least 24 hours.
8. The chest tube is removed when the drainage is less than 150 cc an hour.

COMPLICATIONS

The complication rate with properly performed pleurodesis is low. Transient cough, fever, and pleuritic chest pain are common immediately after the instillation of the sclerosing agents. Pneumothorax is a possible complication with any chest tube insertion and resolves with suction and repositioning the chest tube and dressings. Loculation of the malignant effusion can develop after chest tube insertion by instillation of the sclerosing agent before the lung is reexpanded. Loculation will prevent complete drainage and adequate dispersion of the sclerosing agent. If loculation occurs repositioning the chest tube is not recommended for it may lead to puncture of the lung parenchyma. Empyema and fistula formation can be avoided with sterile technique. If a fistula or sinus tract develops, the area should be cultured and treated with dilute hydrogen peroxide.

Chapter 15

Oncologic Emergencies

HYPERCALCEMIA OF MALIGNANCY

Hypercalcemia, the most common metabolic abnormality observed in cancer patients, generally presents in patients with advanced disease and may occur in the absence of bone metastasis. The pathophysiology remains partially elusive. Malignancy is the most common cause of an elevated serum calcium level in the in-patient setting. The malignancies most commonly associated with hypercalcemia include breast cancer, squamous cell lung cancer, and multiple myeloma. Rarely, hypercalcemia can be observed with lymphomas, hypernephroma, and head and neck cancer.

Pathogenesis

The pathogenesis of hypercalcemia associated with malignancy is diverse and can be explained by three postulated mechanisms. Tumors having a propensity to metastasize to bone (i.e. breast cancer) cause bone destruction possibly mediated by prostaglandin secretion by the invading tumor cells. Other tumors, such as squamous cell cancer of the lung, cause hypercalcemia by releasing humoral mediators, including PTH-related protein modified by expression of interleukin-I, tumor necrosis factor, and transforming growth-factor alpha. Hematologic malignancies (i.e. multiple myeloma) produce osteoclast activating factors (OAF) including lymphotoxins, interleukin-I, and tumor necrosis factor, thereby stimulating osteoclast mediated bone resorption.

Presenting Signs and Symptoms

Since calcium metabolism is ubiquitous throughout the body, hypercalcemia affects multiple organ systems, resulting in cardiac, gastrointestinal and renal dysfunction, although the neuromuscular symptoms generally dominate. The level of the serum calcium at presentation and the rapidity at which this level was achieved determine the severity of the symptoms. Although the initial complaints are nonspecific, the cancer patient with hypercalcemia often presents with a deterioration in mental status, anorexia, and dehydration. The common clinical scenario is the bedridden cancer patient who develops polyuria due to the elevated serum calcium. The elevated calcium impairs the concentrating ability of the kidney, thereby exacerbating the dehydration and causing a vicious cycle. The predominant neuromuscular symptoms include confusion, lethargy, fatigue, and somnolence, although seizure and coma may occur. Prevalent gastrointestinal symptoms include nausea, vomiting, obstipation, and constipation. From a cardiac standpoint, hypercalcemia may cause a range of findings from mild EKG changes to severe ventricular arrhythmias.

Treatment

Due to the non-specific presentation, the diagnosis of hypercalcemia must be entertained in any cancer patient, especially those who have cancers with a tendency for hypercalcemia. Although a number of treatment options are available, the agents chosen should be based upon the pathogenesis of the elevated serum calcium, the severity of the hypercalcemia, renal and liver function, and the aggressiveness with which the patient should be treated.

The general guidelines of treatment include saline volume expansion, diuresis with furosemide, and initiation of an inhibitor of bone resorption (glucocorticoids, calcitonin, mithramycin, etidronate). Since most hypercalcemic patients are dehydrated, saline hydration (200 ml/hr, for example) should be used to restore intravascular volume. The sodium ion also competitively inhibits renal tubular resorption of calcium, resulting in urinary calcium excretion. The calcium level, degree of dehydration, cardiac function, and renal function should direct saline infusion rates. Once the intravascular volume has been restored, low doses of intravenous furosemide increase calcium excretion by preventing its reabsorption in the ascending loop of Henle. Saline infusion with furosemide may result in improvement within twenty-four hours, although the serum calcium rarely normalizes unless the patient presented with mild hypercalcemia. The addition of one of the following inhibitors of osteoclast function may be needed.

Glucocorticoids

Glucocorticoids are presently used for treating hypercalcemia associated with breast cancer and hematologic malignancies. Steroids inhibit gastrointestinal absorption of calcium, prevent OAF release, and may cause lysis of tumor cells. Glucocorticoids are generally used in short-term therapy (prednisone 40–100 mg/d or equivalent dose of hydrocortisone) due to the severe side-effects with chronic use.

Calcitonin

By increasing urinary calcium excretion and inhibiting osteoclast function, calcitonin decreases the serum calcium level within hours of infusion with peak nadir in 1–2 days. The decrease in serum calcium may be transient and mild. Calcitonin is given subcutaneously or intramuscularly at a starting dose of 4 IU/kg every 12 to 24 hours with an increase in the dose after two days, if necessary, to 8 IU/kg every 12 hours. All patients should be skin tested prior to the initiation of therapy.

Mithramycin

Mithramycin is an anti-tumor antibiotic that is toxic to osteoclasts, resulting in normalization of serum calcium levels within 24–48 hours after infusion, with peak effect in 1–2 days. The usual starting dose is 25 micrograms/kg administered as a slow intravenous infusion over two to four hours, which may be repeated after two days. Besides its nephrotoxic effect, mithramycin may cause hepatic toxicity, platelet dysfunction, coagulopathy, and myelosuppression, especially thrombocytopenia, with prolonged use. As a result, mithramycin is recommended in refractory cases of hypercalcemia.

Etidronate

Etidronate, one of the bisphosphonate compounds, is a potent inhibitor of osteoclast function. In the acute setting, etidronate is given intravenously (7.5 mg/kg/d) for three consecutive days with each infusion given over four to six hours with dose adjusted for renal insufficiency. Although fairly new, side effects are minimal and include rare transient increase in serum creatinine. Beneficial results are generally obtained within 24–48 hours.

Gallium Nitrate

An agent that may become popular in the near future is gallium nitrate, an inhibitor of bone resorption. The previously utilized regimen of 5 days of continuous infusion at 100–200 mg/m² per day has been effective in producing normocalcemia and improving duration of response. Currently, dose is 200 mg/m²/day for 5 days or less if calcium level returns to normal.

Summary

The goal of treatment of hypercalcemia associated with malignancy is the resolution of disabling symptoms. This clinical scenario is most commonly seen in refractory and end-stage cancer patients. If intervention with chemotherapy is not a viable option, other agents or combinations of agents may be utilized in an attempt to improve the patient's quality of life. The survival rate for cancer patients with hypercalcemia is poor at approximately 40% at three months.

SUPERIOR VENA CAVA SYNDROME

The superior vena cava syndrome (SVCS), a distinct clinical entity, is generally seen in patients with a malignancy. Until recently, the SVCS required prompt therapeutic intervention to prevent any serious problems. Today, oncologists agree with a more deliberate evaluation that would yield a diagnosis and the optimal choice of therapeutic intervention (chemotherapy and/or radiation therapy).

Etiology

The SVCS includes an insidious onset of progressive erythema and edema of the unilateral upper extremity along with ipsilateral neck and facial involvement. Venous distension is commonly seen on the neck and occasionally on the chest wall due to the formation of venous collateral blood vessels. Cyanosis of the involved extremity is occasionally present. Patients most commonly complain of dyspnea along with edema of the involved extremity, neck, and face.

Understanding the anatomic position of the SVC is important in comprehending the pathogenesis of this syndrome. The SVC is a thin-walled vessel draining venous blood from the upper thorax, upper extremities, head, and neck. Due to its position in the middle mediastinum, any enlargement of the perihilar or paratracheal lymph nodes, or any abnormality of the aorta, pulmonary artery, or large bronchus could lead to impingement upon the SVC. With gradual interruption of the SVC, the azygos vein, an important tributary draining into the SVC, can engorge, enlarge, and form collaterals, thereby allowing bloodflow back to the heart. This also causes the venous engorgement noted on physical exam.

A malignancy, most often of pulmonary primary, especially small cell lung cancer, is the most likely etiology. Other malignancies known to cause SVCS include lymphoma (especially the non-Hodgkin's lymphomas), germ cell tumors, and rarely, other primary or metastatic lesions. Non-malignant etiologies, causing less than 5% of cases of SVCS, include thrombosis involving central venous catheters, pacemakers, aortic aneurysms, mediastinal fibrosis, substernal thyroid, and infectious involvement of the mediastinum.

Workup and Evaluation

In addition to the findings noted on the physical exam, the chest x-ray generally reveals widening of the mediastinum with occasional pleural effusion. A confirmatory thoracic CT may be needed to define the possible etiology (i.e. rule out a lung mass) and to evaluate any critical impingement on important adjacent mediastinal structures. If surgery is contemplated, a venogram would define the extent of anatomic abnormality. A definitive diagnosis should be obtained expeditiously by biopsy of a palpable lymph node, bronchoscopy, thoracentesis, or sputum cytology. If none of the preceding are possible, a mediastinoscopy, thoracotomy, or bone marrow biopsy should be performed.

Treatment

A number of therapeutic options are available, but intervention depends upon the diagnosis obtained through the preceding workup. Small cell lung cancer is treated with combination chemotherapy and localized radiation therapy to the mediastinum. Non-small cell lung cancer is treated with radiation therapy alone. The non-Hodgkin's lymphomas are generally treated with systemic chemotherapy, often with local radiation.

Thrombolytic agents (urokinase, streptokinase) are used in catheter-induced SVCS. In addition to the primary treatment with radiation therapy and/or chemotherapy, supportive measures with low-dose diuretics, supplemental oxygen, and bedrest are also important. Steroids are generally employed (dexamethasone 4–10mg q 6 hrs.) in an attempt to decrease any associated mediastinal edema and inflammation. The dose of radiation is extremely critical. Higher doses (300–400 cGy per treatment) are utilized early in the course of therapy in an attempt to accelerate relief of symptoms. After three to four treatments with this high dose, a lower dose schedule is then employed until 3000–6000 cGy has been given depending upon the histology of the tumor.

Prognosis

The cause of SVCS in the vast majority of patients (>95%) is a malignancy, and this malignancy is most often lung cancer. The prognosis for recovery and survival from the SVCS depends upon the histology and stage of the primary tumor. In general, patients with small cell lung cancer or lymphoma respond well to the combination of chemotherapy and radiation therapy. Unfortunately, those patients with non-small cell lung cancer may respond well initially to radiation therapy, but often their one year survival is less than 20%.

Summary

The superior vena cava syndrome is a distinct clinical entity with unique presenting signs and symptoms. It is imperative to make a tissue diagnosis that will direct optimal therapeutic intervention. The majority of patients with SVCS possess a malignancy most often of lung primary. The recovery from and prognosis of the SVCS is dependent upon the etiology and stage of the primary tumor at the time of presentation.

TUMOR LYSIS SYNDROME

Tumor lysis syndrome (TLS) is a serious metabolic emergency seen in cancer patients with highly chemotherapy-sensitive tumors. It is essential to recognize potential risk factors and early signs of TLS since prophylactic intervention could prevent life-threatening consequences.

Etiology

TLS is generally seen in malignancies with rapid proliferative rates, such as aggressive lymphomas, acute leukemias and, rarely, solid tumors. The clinical scenario consists of the rapid onset of hyperkalemia, hyperuricemia, and hyperphosphatemia with hypocalcemia after the initiation of chemotherapy. There have been rare reports of TLS occurring after the initiation of glucocorticoids or radiation therapy. Antecedent risk factors include high tumor bulk (i.e. numerous sites of disease or large mass of tumor), elevated uric acid, elevated lactate dehydrogenase and azotemia with oliguria.

Pathogenesis

The onset of TLS can occur within hours of initiation of chemotherapy and be prolonged over the course of days during cell breakdown. The sudden lysis of tumor cells rapidly causes hyperkalemia and hyperphosphatemia.

Hyperkalemia

The hyperkalemia of TLS is due to the cytotoxic effects of chemotherapy, although ensuing renal insufficiency exacerbates the degree of hyperkalemia. The pseudo-hyperkalemia occasionally seen with leukocytosis and thrombocytosis must always be considered. The resulting hyperkalemia may result in neuromuscular manifestations (paresthesias, weakness, and areflexia) along with severe cardiac manifestations, including cardiac arrest.

Hyperphosphatemia

The rapid onset of the elevated serum phosphate levels is also the result of cell lysis. The resulting hyperphosphatemia can cause metastatic calcification within soft tissues (i.e. renal tubules) especially if the calcium-phosphate product is greater than sixty.

Hyperuricemia

The breakdown of intracellular nucleic acids by xanthine oxidase yields hyperuricemia. The increased serum uric acid concentration may cause urate nephropathy with renal insufficiency and sudden attacks of gouty arthritis. As will be described, the main emphasis of treatment of TLS is an attempt at preventing uric acid nephropathy.

Hypocalcemia

The hypocalcemia, a direct result of the hyperphosphatemia and metastatic calcification, is generally mild, and symptoms are rare. Progressive and persistent hypocalcemia may result in neuromuscular manifestations including circumoral paresthesias, carpopedal spasm (Trousseau's sign), and neuromuscular irritability (Chvostek's sign) with more severe symptoms, including deterioration in mental status, seizures, or convulsions.

Treatment

The main emphasis on treatment of TLS is recognition of predisposing risk factors and prevention. Due to the serious nature of the metabolic derangements, close monitoring of daily renal function and metabolites, including potassium, calcium, phosphorus, and uric acid is essential. The major emphasis of intervention is an attempt to prevent renal damage secondary to the hyperuricemia.

One to two days prior to the initiation of chemotherapy, *saline hydration* should be initiated to achieve adequate urine output (4–5 litres/d) during chemotherapy. Due to the high fluid rate, strict attention should be placed upon daily weights, intake and output. *Allopurinol* should be initiated, with the starting dose dependent upon the serum uric acid level. Elevated dosages (i.e. 300 mg TID) may be used acutely with rapid taper to maintenance dose (100–300 mg/d) after two to three days of therapy. By decreasing the formation of uric acid, allopurinol should decrease the incidence of uric acid nephropathy. Due to its renal excretion, the allopurinol dose should be adjusted in patients with renal insufficiency. *Alkalinization* of the urine may also lead to increased excretion of uric acid. If the urine pH < 7, sodium bicarbonate should be added to the infusing intravenous fluid. Alkalinization should be avoided if hyperphosphatemia is present, since alkaline urine can initiate renal tubular calcium-phosphate precipitation.

The *hyperkalemia* associated with TLS can be sudden, severe and life-threatening. If EKG changes are present, careful infusion of calcium should be given while the patient is on a cardiac monitor. This needs to be done cautiously since an elevated phosphate level may lead to metastatic calcification. Other available agents include intravenous glucose with insulin, and intravenous bicarbonate although cation exchange resins offer removal of potassium from the body.

The *hyperphosphatemia* can be easily managed with oral phosphate-binders to decrease absorption and saline diuresis to aid in phosphate excretion. By an unknown mechanism, the diuretic acetazolamide inhibits proximal tubular reabsorption of phosphates and also contributes to urine alkalinization.

Summary

Tumor lysis syndrome is seen in rapidly growing, chemotherapy-sensitive tumors. The recognition of predisposing risk factors and rapid therapeutic intervention may prevent any serious consequences. It is important to consider the role of dialysis in patients with persistent and progressive fluid overload, hyperkalemia (>6 meq/l), hyperuricemia (>10 mg/dl), and/or hyperphosphatemia (10 mg/dl).

SPINAL CORD COMPRESSION

Spinal cord compression is an acute medical emergency. Forewarning signs and symptoms allow early therapeutic intervention, thereby preventing progressive or irreversible neurological deterioration. The severity of neurological impairment at presentation dictates the potential reversibility of symptoms.

Etiology

Although spinal cord compression can result from either a primary spinal cord tumor or metastatic lesion, the latter are more common and generally involve the vertebral body. The expanding metastatic focus within the bony vertebrae may impinge upon the anterior aspect of the spinal cord, yielding neurological signs and symptoms. Some tumors (lymphoma and seminoma) may arise in a paraspinal position and invade inward into the vertebral foramen, thereby imposing on neural elements. Involvement of the spinal cord neural elements below L1-L2 comprises the cauda equina syndrome.

Spinal cord compression is most common with tumors that have a tendency to metastasize to bone, especially lung cancer, breast cancer, prostate cancer, and multiple myeloma. The distribution of involvement includes the cervical vertebrae (10%), thoracic vertebrae (70%), and lumbosacral vertebrae (20%). The upper thoracic vertebrae comprise the most crucial area of involvement due to the degree of confinement and the tenuous blood supply. The lumbosacral vertebrae are the preferable sites of metastasis for gastrointestinal malignancies.

Presenting Signs and Symptoms

Pain, the most common preliminary symptom, may be localized or radicular and precedes the onset of further neurologic deterioration by weeks to months. *Motor loss* and *weakness* of the involved extremities (i.e. quadraparesis with a cervical lesion or paraparesis with a lower thoracic or lumbosacral lesion) with *sensory loss* follows. Patients often describe an ascending tingling sensation beginning in the distal extremities. *Autonomic dysfunction*, a late manifestation, involves urinary and gastrointestinal systems and causes loss of bowel or bladder control, urinary retention, and constipation. Once motor loss and weakness develop, neurologic deterioration may be rapid and, sometimes, irreversible.

Physical Exam

The physical exam often reveals tenderness over the vertebrae. Pain localized with movement may pinpoint the involved vertebrae. The neurologic exam may reveal signs consistent with an upper motor neuron lesion, such as weakness, spasticity, hyperreflexia, and the presence of abnormal reflexes (e.g. Babinski's sign). Sensory findings are generally evident below the level of spinal cord involvement and most marked distally. Often, a sensory level may be detected. If autonomic dysfunction is suspected, decreased rectal tone and a distended bladder may be noted. The cauda equina syndrome, a term used to explain nerve involvement below the area of L1-L2 nerve roots, is characterized by findings consistent with a lower motor neuron lesion. The exam may yield flaccid areflexia with asymmetrical paraparesis and sensory loss in a saddle distribution up to L1. Pain is commonly present in the perineal area and thighs.

Workup and Evaluation

Spinal cord compression generally occurs in a patient with known cancer and rarely, occurs as the initial presenting complaint. It may be the first evidence of metastatic disease in a patient with a history of cancer. Routine blood work may reveal an elevated *alkaline phosphatase* indicating involvement of bone. *Plain radiographs* of the entire spine should be obtained promptly, with attention to the area of pain noted on the physical exam. Abnormalities on the plain film suggestive of bone involvement include compression or destruction of a vertebral body, or loss of a transverse or spinous process. There may be evidence of lytic or blastic lesions. The majority of patients have bone abnormalities on plain film. The standard test for diagnosing spinal cord compression has been the *myelogram with metrizamide*, a water soluble agent. A lumbar puncture is performed in the L1-L2 area. After removal of fluid for the preliminary studies (protein, glucose, and cytology), metrizamide is injected into the dural sac surrounding the spinal cord. An area of abrupt demarcation pinpoints the area of cord compression. It is imperative to evaluate the extent of the block with either a *C1-C2 puncture* or *CT scan* after the metrizamide injection. The *MRI*, a noninvasive manner of obtaining sagittal and transverse images of the spinal cord, may distinguish the exact location of the lesion in relation to the spinal cord.

Treatment

Once the physical exam is completed and the diagnosis of spinal cord compression acknowledged, the patient should immediately be started on steroids, although controversy exists concerning dose. A common regimen is dexamethasone at 10 mg IVP at presentation followed by 16 mg/day in divided doses. If high-dose steroids are preferred, dexamethasone should be initiated at 100 mg/d in four doses for three days with a rapid taper over two weeks. Although there may be no change in neurologic outcome with high-dose steroids, rapid relief of pain is often noted.

Treatment options include radiation therapy, surgery, chemotherapy, or a combination of the three. A common treatment includes the initiation of steroids with high-dose radiation therapy (300–400 cGy per day for 3 days). The total radiation dose is 3000–4000 cGy over 4–5 weeks with radiation fields extending two vertebral bodies above and below the involved vertebrae. In the acute setting, surgery is an alternative in patients with evidence of spinal instability or if tissue diagnosis is needed. Other indications for surgery include progression of neurologic deficits while receiving radiation therapy, relapse at a site of previous radiation, or the presence of an abscess or hematoma as the etiologic factor. Surgery is followed by radiation therapy due to the difficulty in removing all of the tumor during the procedure. Chemotherapy is generally utilized in combination with one of the other modalities.

Prognosis

In general, slowly progressive neurologic symptoms are associated with a better outcome than are rapidly progressive symptoms. The prognosis of the patient correlates with the severity of neurologic deterioration at presentation. The great majority of patients presenting with paraplegia do not become ambulatory after treatment. Although paraparesis and sensory involvement are a concern, some patients regain function after treatment. After stabilization of disease, the initiation of physical therapy is critical.

Summary

Spinal cord compression is an acute medical emergency with preceding signs and symptoms requiring early recognition to prevent progressive and irreversible neurological deficits. Expedient intervention is necessary with the choice of therapeutic options dictated by the clinical scenario. The degree of neurological impairment at presentation determines potential reversibility of symptoms. The best neurologic result is achieved when pain is the only symptom at presentation.

CARCINOMATOUS MENINGITIS

Carcinomatous meningitis, an uncommon form of metastatic systemic cancer, is an oncologic emergency since progressive neurological disease and death may occur within 4–6 weeks if not treated. Although the true incidence of carcinomatous meningitis is not known, many oncologists note an increased incidence due to the prolonged lifespans of cancer patients and improved chemotherapy. Due to the difficulty in establishing the diagnosis and the poor prognosis often achieved with therapy, carcinomatous meningitis is a frustrating disorder.

Incidence and Traits

Approximately 15% of all cancer patients have neurological signs and symptoms related to their disease, though less than 5% of all primary cancers arise in the central nervous system. Many malignancies metastasize to the CNS, most commonly, lung cancer, breast cancer, and melanoma, with adenocarcinoma as the most common histology. Other malignancies that commonly cause either parenchymal or leptomeningeal metastases include leukemias, lymphomas, gastrointestinal, and genitourinary cancers. The incidence of carcinomatous meningitis due to hematological malignancies, such as leukemia and lymphoma, is decreasing due to CNS prophylaxis with intrathecal chemotherapy and/or cranial irradiation.

Signs and Symptoms

Diagnosing carcinomatous meningitis (CM) can be difficult, requiring clinical signs and symptoms supported by laboratory tests that often have a low sensitivity. The majority of patients have a prior history of cancer, although rarely, CM may rarely be the presenting sign.

At the time of diagnosis of CM, the leptomeninges are diffusely involved throughout the neuraxis. The diffuse involvement results in a variety of clinical presentations. The tumor may obstruct CSF flow resulting in headache, nausea, vomiting, and a deterioration in mental status. The physical exam may reveal papilledema, paresis, or seizure activity. The diagnosis may be confirmed with a head CT scan revealing hydrocephalus. The nerve roots can be involved as they traverse the subarachnoid space resulting in weakness, paresthesias, neck and back pain, or cranial nerve findings. Local CNS involvement from metastatic disease may result in focal findings on exam or a change in mental status. Due to the diversity of presentation, the diagnosis of CM must be considered in any cancer patient presenting with a constellation of neurologic abnormalities.

Diagnosis

The clinical presentation of a cancer patient with new neurological signs and symptoms should be extensively and cautiously evaluated. If CM is a concern, a lumbar puncture should be performed after a head CT scan has ruled out a mass lesion. The findings consistent with CM include an elevated CSF pressure, elevated protein level, and decreased glucose level. The CSF may reveal an increased number of lymphocytes as a reaction to inflammation. The sensitivity of detecting malignant cells within the CSF ranges from 25% to 50%. The first CSF sample yields 50%–60% sensitivity with 4% false positives. The sensitivity rises to 90% with three samples of CSF. As a result, the absence of malignant cells within the CSF does not exclude the diagnosis of CM since malignant cells appear most commonly with widespread meningeal involvement.

Computed tomography and myelography may be useful in establishing the diagnosis of CM. The head CT scan may reveal suggestions of CSF obstruction with enlargement of the ventricles and hydrocephalus. Head CT scan findings consistent with subdural hematoma with a follow-up biopsy revealing dural carcinomatosis have been reported. The myelogram may reveal nodularity of nerve roots resulting in irregularities of the subarachnoid space. The role of MRI with gadolinium is presently being evaluated.

Treatment

CM is commonly treated with a combination of CNS radiation and intrathecal chemotherapy. Once the diagnosis of CM is confirmed, radiation is delivered to the area of CNS with most involvement. A patient with progressive lower extremity weakness may receive radiation to the lumbosacral spine. Since high doses of systemic chemotherapy are needed, intrathecal chemotherapy is preferred, with cytarabine or methotrexate commonly used. During the course of radiation, the patient may have surgical placement of an Omaya reservoir allowing direct access to cerebral ventricles and CSF. The Omaya reservoir, a subcutaneous depot located on the scalp, allows quick and easy access to CSF with the benefit of achieving high CSF drug concentrations with minimal systemic effects. A combination of radiation (2400 cGy) followed by intrathecal methotrexate twice weekly for two weeks is often used. Depending upon clinical improvement and CSF evaluation, intrathecal methotrexate may then be given every one to four weeks. Citrovorum factor may be added orally or intravenously, to prevent the systemic side-effects of methotrexate, which may include stomatitis and myeloid suppression.

During therapy, the patient's CSF should be obtained prior to each intrathecal administration and monitored for the presence of malignant cells, glucose level, and protein level. In general, the propensity for stabilization or improvement is dependent upon the severity of the initial neurological signs. Unfortunately, even with treatment, CM often carries grave prognosis. Untreated, death may occur within 4–6 weeks.

Complications

Complications of therapy may be due to the instillation of intrathecal chemotherapy, radiation, and the use of the Omaya reservoir. The mild nausea, vomiting, and fatigue with radiation is limited if steroids are given concomitantly. The systemic effects of intrathecal chemotherapy are generally minimal, although myelosuppression should be monitored. The intrathecal injection rarely causes arachnoiditis, neurological toxicity (motor deficits, paresis), aseptic meningitis, meningoencephalitis or leukencephalopathy. Although unusual, the most common problems associated with the Omaya reservoir include misplacement, infection and hematoma.

Summary

The diagnosis of CM is based upon clinical presentation with diffuse involvement of the neuraxis, along with occasional isolation of malignant cells within the CSF. Although CM carries a grave prognosis, treatment can be instituted with radiation and intrathecal chemotherapy, thereby relieving disabling symptoms. Sensitive tests must be developed to localize malignant cells within the CSF and to optimize therapy.

Chapter 16

Health Insurance and the Cancer Patient

A MAJOR PROBLEM FOR MANY CANCER PATIENTS

The adequacy of insurance coverage is a major problem for many people who have had a cancer diagnosis at any time in their lives. On diagnosis of the disease, some patients face the loss of, or a reduction in, insurance coverage. Some cancel their policies because the diagnosis triggers a steep rise in premiums. Some patients remain married to a spouse whose insurance covers them or stay in a particular job in order to retain coverage when they would not otherwise choose to. Adolescents whose cancer treatment is covered under a parental subscriber may lose benefits on reaching adulthood and find it difficult to obtain coverage in their own names. Some people who are receiving Welfare and Medicaid benefits remain unemployed rather than lose the Medicaid coverage that comes along with Welfare.

The typical lifetime hospitalization benefit of most comprehensive insurance plans is $500,000. This amount ought to cover a few hospitalizations adequately, but obtaining individual insurance coverage after using up this benefit is difficult and expensive. Policies for high-risk individuals tend to require high premiums.

Discrimination

The problem of insurance discrimination against persons who have had a cancer diagnosis has not yet been thoroughly explored and described. Insurance companies base their rates on actuarial statistics in order to remain viable, and it is legal for them to vary the cost of premiums in accordance with the varying health risk factors of particular populations. However, some cancer patients have reported instances of what they consider undue discrimination.

It has been claimed that some employers have forced cancer patients to give up their group health insurance coverage in order to retain their jobs. The manager of a small company might do this because companies with fewer than 25 employees may not be able to get group insurance coverage if one of those employees has a history of cancer. Companies with only 25 to 100 employees may also be required by their health insurance company to limit coverage of pre-existing conditions. Large companies have tended to have few or no limits and need ask no medical questions when a new employee is added to the group health plan. Some small businesses band together within the Small Business Association in order to take advantage of better rates as an aggregate.

Legal Rights

The Rehabilitation Act of 1973 (Public Law 93-112) applies to persons having or regarded as having substantial impairments and includes cancer patients and persons with a history of cancer. This law prohibits discrimination against the handicapped by entities receiving financial assistance from the U.S. Department of Health and Human Services. Complaints related to this law can be filed with the Office of Civil Rights, Department of Health and Human Services.

Insurance companies are regulated at the state level, and state laws vary. The laws address rates, policy conditions, termination or reinstatement of coverage, and the scope of coverage and benefits. All states have insurance commissions or departments that enforce state laws regarding the types of coverage that must be available and when rates may be increased. The insurance commissions, which mediate between the insurance companies and the citizens of the state according to the state government's concepts of the benefit of the state as a whole, have a great deal of influence in situations of conflict. Patients who have been treated unfairly by an insurance company may contact their state's insurance commission for information on the laws governing insurance in their state and to complain about their situation. American Cancer Society brochure 45585-PS lists agencies to which complaints may be addressed. If an insurance company refuses to provide reimbursement for necessary and appropriate treatment within the coverage of the patient's policy, the patient may retain a lawyer and sue for non-coverage. Often, a compromise or exception is then negotiated for the patient.

COBRA (Consolidated Omnibus Budget Reconciliation Act of 1986) is a federal law that requires employers to offer group health insurance to employees and their dependents who lose their regular group coverage due to individual circumstances, such as leaving the company, being fired, or working fewer hours. All employers of more than 20 employees must provide for continuation of insurance coverage in such cases and must include surviving, divorced, or separated spouses and dependent children. Continued group coverage is extended for 18 months for the employee and for 36 months for spouses and dependents at rates that are usually higher than group rates but may not exceed a particular limit. The employer must offer continued coverage regardless of any pre-existing conditions, including cancer.

Options and Recommendations for the Patient

Patients shopping for health insurance should carefully compare policies regarding fee schedules for various procedures and services, the way in which claims are processed, and what is covered in any of the states in which they will be treated. Your local office of the American Cancer Society may be able to provide information on cancer-related aspects of various insurance companies' policies.

In general, group insurance provides lower rates than does individual insurance. Patients who are members of professional or social organizations may have access to "guaranteed issue" plans. Employees of large companies are often guaranteed participation in a group plan in spite of previous diagnoses. Health maintenance organizations (HMOs) offer comprehensive coverage, and many allow anyone to enroll during an annual open enrollment period.

Comprehensive Health Care (CHC) plans, which must accept high-risk applicants, generally cover all costs of health care and spread the risk of covering high-risk individuals among a state's health insurance companies. They are generally less expensive than private high-risk plans. Premiums vary widely among the several states that have implemented CHC plans, but all tend to be high.

Special cancer-oriented insurance policies often have hidden limitations and have been evaluated by the U.S. House Select Committee on Aging as not cost-effective for the elderly, in particular, and several states have banned their sale.

Hospital indemnity plans, offered through large companies and clubs via direct mail, can be purchased to supplement a patient's basic medical insurance. Most require a one-year waiting period for pre-existing conditions but cover other claims immediately.

Medicare covers most people age 65 or older as well as younger people who are disabled and have been receiving Social Security disability benefits for approximately two years. Patients who do not have enough medical insurance—or none at all—may be eligible for Medicaid, and Medicaid and other state and local benefits may be available to low-income or unemployed persons.

Patients must get approval from many insurance companies for any nonemergency hospital admission. It is important for patients to know the limits of their insurance coverage for both in-patient and out-patient treatment. Because insurance companies change policies and interpretations of guidelines over time and exercise some judgment on a case-by-case basis, patients should contact their insurance companies to discuss their particular situations. Patients enrolling in clinical studies should be sure to check with the treatment team to see which parts of treatment will be free-of-charge and which parts they must pay for.

Contrary to the expectations of many cancer patients and survivors, life insurance is also available to most, though the price may be high. If the person's survival prognosis is good, a reasonable rate may be available.

Each Division of the American Cancer Society is equipped with resource materials to help in answering questions or providing referral to appropriate help. For a free copy of the brochure "Cancer, Your Job, Insurance, and the Law," a patient may contact his or her local office of the American Cancer Society. The National Cancer Employment Law (NCEL) Project has been compiling information for the ACS on laws and administrative and court decisions pertaining to employment and disability. The NCEL is also serving as a resource for legislative initiatives to promote reintegration of the cancer survivor in the work force and to reduce employment discrimination encountered by cancer survivors.

Recommendations for the House Officer

Credit policies vary widely among healthcare institutions (even between hospitals and associated clinics); it can't be assumed that all "medically necessary" treatment costs will be covered by insurance or, failing this, will be absorbed by the hospital. Local implementation of private and government-subsidized insurance may also have a large financial impact on patients. Medicare insurance generally covers perhaps forty percent of healthcare costs, not one hundred percent, and many patients do not purchase supplemental insurance to fill in the gap. The costs of some tests may be much greater than one would expect, and the total cost of care ruinous to the patient who "spends down" (depending on the vagaries of insurance and credit policies), so it is wise to find out local costs and reimbursement practices and, when in doubt, to enquire.

Because many insurance companies now require that the patient receive prior approval before any hospital stay except in cases of extreme emergency, your hospital business office assesses the patient's insurance coverage during pre-admission screening. In many hospitals, the business office then contacts the utilization review department, which obtains the insurer's approval for the admission. When you are writing chart notes, stay in touch with your hospital's utilization review department so that documention is appropriate and timely in order to ensure all legitimate reimbursement. Appropriate documentation is also important to support cases reviewed retrospectively. If the insurance company says that the hospital should have notified the patient that the insurance would not cover the admission, there are financial repercussions on the hospital and credibility is impaired, making it harder to negotiate reimbursement in the future. Some insurance companies now employ case managers, generally registered nurses, to make recommendations about treatment that may need to be reconciled with your decisions through your utilization review department. Sometimes, case managers introduce helpful flexibility into the interpretation of benefits and funding of traditionally non-covered alternatives to hospitalization.

Definitions of reasonable and necessary treatment have shifted over the years. Knowing the costs of various tests at your institution can help you assess the appropriate frequency for them relative to the benefit they yield. Even at health maintenance organizations, it is important to ensure that your business office can justify a particular outpatient treatment if you want to ensure reimbursement. If the medical literature with which you are familiar indicates that a particular treatment, such as a chemo-therapeutic agent, may be effective in your patient's situation, and this use of the drug is not indicated on an FDA label, an insurance company may consider that use of the drug experimental and, therefore, nonreimbursable. Local Blue Cross/Blue Shield plans, however, have recently started to evaluate drugs themselves instead of relying solely on FDA label indications. The Association of Community Cancer Centers (ACCC), which has been studying this issue and reimbursement for experimental therapies, may be able to offer you guidance in particular cases if your hospital is a member institution or through the quarterly publication Oncology Issues. You can contact Lee Mortenson, M.S, M.P.A., Executive Director, ACCC, at 11600 Nebel Street, Suite 201, Rockville, Maryland 20852; (301) 984-9496.

In situations in which treatment is unusual or difficult for the patient to explain, or if the patient has trouble gaining reimbursement from the insurance company, you may assist the patient by contacting the insurance company's medical director on a physician-to-physician basis. In some cases, insurance companies have changed their reimbursement practices after discussions of the medical issues. If an insurance company refuses reimbursement for treatment that is proper in your medical judgment, and you fail to protest the limitation of coverage, you may be liable in a lawsuit if the patient is harmed by lack of the treatment. If you protest, and the insurance company still refuses reimbursement due to defects in the design or implementation of cost containment mechanisms and this is determined to have resulted in a medically inappropriate decision, the insurer may be held legally liable. Your hospital quality assurance, utilization review, or peer review organization may be able to assist you if such a situation arises.

Your hospital social worker or hospital patient accounting department can assist you by explaining issues related to insurance coverage to the patient and advocating with the insurance company on behalf of a patient. If the process of intervening with an insurance company becomes overly time-consuming, consider requesting the assistance of your hospital administration.

Chapter 17

Cancer-Related Information for Your Patients

There are many sources of information to assist the physician in communicating with cancer patients. Among them are the following nationwide organizations that offer books, pamphlets, posters, and other audiovisual materials. There may also be programs and organizations specific to your state or locality. For information on local resources, contact your hospital social worker, your local division of the American Cancer Society, or your local library's reference desk.

The American Cancer Society (ACS). This organization of volunteers is dedicated to controlling and eradicating cancer. The ACS offers a basic descriptive booklet ("American Cancer Society: What It Is, What It Does, How It Began, Who Directs It, Where It Is Going") describing its programs in public and professional education, service to patients and families, and research.

The society is organized in 58 divisions, one in each state, one in Puerto Rico, one in the District of Columbia, and six others in metropolitan areas, each listed in the White Pages of telephone books. Contact your local office of the ACS for most publications. National headquarters are at 1599 Clifton Road, N.E., Altanta, Georgia 30329; telephone (404) 320-3333.

The ACS publishes literature and audio-visual materials on cancer prevention, risk reduction, detection, and other aspects of cancer, some in other languages. For a list of materials ("Request Form for Adult Cancer Education Programs"), contact your local office of the American Cancer Society. The ACS also disseminates information about cancer and ACS support services to the public via its Cancer Response System at (800) ACS-2345. A list of "Coast to Coast Cancer Camps" is available from the System. Information on questionable treatment methods is available from the ACS Office of Unproven Methods at (404) 320-3333. *Cancer Facts and Figures* is an annual publication of the American Cancer Society. It provides statistics based on the SEER (Surveillance, Epidemiology, and End Results) program on selected cancer sites and on cancer by age and race in the U.S. and Puerto Rico. "Cancer Statistics" is published as the January/February issue of *CA—A Cancer Journal for Clinicians, a Journal of the American Cancer Society.* It contains information on cancer incidence, survival, and mortality for the United States and around the world, prepared by the ACS Department of Epidemiology and Statistics. You may also find the *ACS Professional Education Materials Catalog* helpful.

The Association for Brain Tumor Research, 3725 N. Talman Avenue, Chicago, Illinois 60618, (312) 286-5571, is a voluntary, not-for-profit organization supporting research on and promoting the understanding of brain tumors. The Association publishes pamphlets and booklets on types of tumors and treatment modalities, as well as a descriptive pamphlet about the organization itself.

Cancer Care, Inc., 1180 Avenue of the Americas, New York, NY 10036, (212) 221-3300, is the service arm of the National Cancer Foundation, an organization that provides professional counseling and planning for advanced cancer patients and their families. Cancer Care is a not-for-profit social service agency that helps patients and families cope with the emotional, psychological, and financial consequences of cancer in all stages of the illness. The organization offers home visits by trained volunteers, counseling, literature, referral, work site advocacy, financial assistance for non-medical expenses, and home care planning. Publications of Cancer Care include a "Guide to Services" pamphlet, a card about the organization's answer line, and the booklet "What About Me? A Booklet for Teenage Children of Cancer Patients."

Candlelighters Childhood Cancer Foundation, Inc., 1312 18th St., N.W., 2nd Floor, Washington, D.C. 20036, (202) 659-5136, is a nonprofit, international network of mutual support and education groups for parents of children with cancer. Candlelighters also offers groups for teenage cancer patients and teenage siblings of children who have cancer. The Metropolitan Washington Candlelighters group is a registered lobbyist, coordinating congressional testimony and monitoring federal programs affecting families of children with cancer. Candlelighters produces many publications, including periodicals, described in the foundation's "Publications List" and "Basic Family Library" brochure.

CanSurmount, New York, NY, (212) 382-2169, is a program of the ACS that is available from some but not all local units of the ACS. CanSurmount offers patient and family visitation, with the physician's awareness and approval, by volunteers who have had cancer and who are carefully selected and specially trained to provide emotional support and information on community resources to cancer patients. Whenever possible, the volunteer is matched with the patient for similarity in cancer diagnosis, age, sex, and socioeconomic status. CanSurmount is described briefly in the ACS booklet and in more depth in a print-out from the ACS Cancer Response System.

Concern for Dying, 250 W. 57th Street, Room 831, New York, NY 10107, (212) 246-6962, is a nonprofit educational council that provides information about living wills, maintains a Living Will Registry, disseminates advice on legal questions related to patients' rights, sponsors a collaborative network within which healthcare professionals can address issues related to the terminally ill, and gives assistance to families of the terminally ill in instances of institutional reluctance to honor patients' wishes. Concern for Dying offers publications and audio-visual materials related to these topics.

Corporate Angel Network, Inc. (CAN), Westchester County Airport, Building One, White Plains, New York 10604, (914) 328-1313. This nonprofit, nationwide organization finds space on corporate airplane flights for cancer patients who need transportation to treatment centers. Referrals are accepted from social service and medical personnel, family members, or friends, but CAN must speak directly with the patient or person traveling with the patient in order to explain the program. Requests for transportation are taken when a definite date for an appointment or discharge has been made, not more than three weeks in advance. A printed description of the organization and requirements for traveling patients is available on request from the Network headquarters office.

Encore, National Board YWCA, 726 Broadway, New York, NY 10003, is a national program of the Young Women's Christian Association (YWCA), providing an exercise plan and discussion group for postoperative breast cancer patients. Contact your local YWCA to see whether the program is available in your area. A descriptive brochure is available from the New York office.

I Can Cope is an eight-week series of two-hour classes presented by community professionals and sponsored by the ACS, often in cooperation with local hospitals or health agencies. The program provides information on cancer biology and research, diagnosis, treatment, side effects, and nutrition and other aspects of daily living, as well as encouragement and referral to local resources. The program, designed for cancer patients and their families, is free. Contact your local ACS office for more information. The program is described briefly in the ACS booklet and in more depth in a print-out from the ACS Cancer Response System.

The International Association of Laryngectomees (some local chapters are called Lost Cord Clubs, New Voice Clubs, or Anamilo) is an ACS program of volunteers who visit patients and offer speech training and support to persons who have lost their voices to cancer. The association maintains a registry of postlaryngectomy speech instructors and publishes educational materials. The program is described briefly in the ACS booklet and in more depth in a print-out from the ACS Cancer Response System.

Leukemia Society of America, 733 Third Avenue, New York, NY 10017, (212) 573-8484, has local chapters listed in the White Pages of telephone books. The society's Family Support Groups help patients, families, and friends deal with leukemia, lymphoma, Hodgkin's disease, and multiple myeloma and provide up to $750 worth of financial assistance to patients with leukemia, lymphoma, and Hodgkin's disease for drugs, laboratory costs associated with transfusions, transportation, and radiation therapy. The society produces publications and audio-visual materials on many aspects of this group of diseases, some of them in Spanish as well as English, and several of them addressing children's concerns. A newsletter is also published by the headquarters office.

Living Bank, P.O. Box 6725, Houston, Texas 77265, operates a registry and referral service for people who want to make a commitment to donating their tissues, bones, or vital organs to transplantation or research. Living Bank also informs the public about organ donation and transplantation. The organization's toll-free telephone number is (800) 528-2971. It is also described in a print-out from the ACS Cancer Response System.

Look Good . . . Feel Better is a nationwide, community-based public service program developed by the Cosmetic, Toiletry and Fragrance Association (CTFA) and available through the ACS and the National Cosmetology Association. The program provides an opportunity for people undergoing cancer treatment to have a no-cost visit with a specially trained cosmetology professional who focuses on beauty techniques to help patients maintain their appearance while undergoing chemotherapy or radiation therapy. A booklet of tips and the locations of participating salons are available via the toll-free telephone number (800) 558-5005.

Make-A-Wish Foundation of America, 4601 North 16th Street, Suite 205, Phoenix, Arizona 85016, is a foundation that works closely with the families of children up to the age of eighteen who have terminal illnesses to grant a special wish of the child. The foundation covers all expenses involved in granting the wish and arranges for all details involved, including transportation, if needed. You can call the foundation toll-free at (800) 722-9474. An annual report, a pamphlet, and other descriptive materials are available from the headquarters office.

Make Today Count, Inc. (MTC), 101 1/2 S. Union Street, Alexandria, Virginia 22314, (703) 548-9674, is a nonprofit organization offering emotional support to persons with cancer and other life-threatening illnesses and to their family members, friends, and the professionals who work with them. MTC offers a newsletter and has published the books *Make Today Count* and *Until Tomorrow Comes*.

The National Cancer Institute (NCI), is a part of the National Institutes of Health, which is administered by the U.S. Department of Health and Human Services and is supported by annual appropriations from Congress. The NCI provides pamphlets for patients and laymen discussing different types and sites of cancer, early detection, treatment, and research reports. Contact the National Cancer Institute's **Cancer Information Service** free-of-charge by calling (800) 4-CANCER; in Alaska, call (800) 638-6694; in Hawaii, call 524-1234 on Oahu, collect from neighbor islands. Some pamphlets are available in other languages; all NCI publications are free. Quantities may be ordered from the NCI Office of Cancer Communications, Building 31, Room 10A24, Bethesda, Maryland 20892. The NCI's "Publications List for the Public and Patients" describes these publications and provides an order blank. The NCI also sponsors Physician's Data Query (PDQ), a database of the most current and effective treatments for cancer patients, clinical studies currently under way, and physicians and institutions with a major interest in cancer. Patients have access to PDQ and other informational resources of the NCI by calling the Cancer Information Service.

The National Charities Information Bureau, Inc., 19 Union Square W., New York, NY 10003-3395, (212) 929-6300, publishes standards for, and information on, the conduct of charitable organizations, including those relevant to cancer. Their "Wise Giving Guide" lists charities and characterizes their practices.

The National Coalition for Cancer Survivorship (NCCS), 323 Eighth St. SW, Albuquerque, NM 87102, (505) 764-9956, is a network of organizations and individuals concerned with the quality of life after a person receives a diagnosis of cancer. The organization also works to reduce cancer-based discrimination in employment and insurance and serves as a national voice for cancer survivors in the media, government, and health communities. Through the *NCCS Networker* newsletter and speakers, the NCCS communicates that survivors can live vibrant and productive lives.

The National Hospice Organization (NHS), 1901 N. Moore Street, Suite 901, Arlington, Virginia 22209, (703) 243-5900, is a nonprofit organization of groups providing hospice care and concerned with care of the terminally ill and their families. NHS provides literature, information, and referral to local hospice programs and regional and national resources and runs a hospice career placement listing service.

The Ostomy Rehabilitation Program of the ACS gives psychological support and encourages the training of enterostomal therapists who work with patients in adjusting bodily functions to daily living. For more information, contact your local office of the ACS. The program is described briefly in the ACS booklet and in more depth in a print-out from the ACS Cancer Response System.

The Philanthropic Advisory Service of the Council of Better Business Bureaus, Inc. (CBBB), 4200 Wilson Boulevard, Suite 80, Arlington, Virginia 22203, (703) 276-0100, publishes standards and provides information on the practices of charitable organizations, including those related to cancer. The service also educates donors about charitable giving. "Give, But Give Wisely," a bi-monthly list of charities generating the most inquiries to the service, summarizes which ones do and don't meet CBBB standards.

Reach to Recovery, a program of the ACS, provides temporary prostheses when needed, teaches post-surgery exercises, and provides visitation and counseling to aid breast cancer patients in returning to normal lives. For more information, contact your local office of the ACS. The program is described briefly in the ACS booklet and in more depth in a print-out from the ACS Cancer Response System.

Road to Recovery is an ACS program that provides transportation for cancer patients to their treatments and home again. Transportation may be provided by volunteer drivers or through reimbursement to paid providers, depending on the resources available in the community. Details are available from local ACS offices. The program is described briefly in the ACS booklet and in more depth in a print-out from the ACS Cancer Response System.

Ronald McDonald Houses, % Golin/Harris Communications, 500 N. Michigan Avenue, Suite 200, Chicago, Illinois 60611, (312) 836-7100, are locally owned and operated, not-for-profit, no- or low-cost homes-away-from home for families of children being treated for serious illness. More than 120 of these houses have been established in North America for the families of seriously ill children being treated at nearby hospitals. Children who are outpatients also stay at the houses with their families. Full-time house managers and volunteers from the community help the families feel at home and cope with the illness and treatment experience. Contact your hospital social worker for information on whether there is a Ronald McDonald House or equivalent near your hospital. Informational materials are available from Golin/Harris Communications.

United Ostomy Association, Inc., 36 Executive Park, Suite 120, Irvine, CA 92714, (714) 660-8624, is a not-for-profit mutual support and educational organization for persons who have ostomies. Local chapters conduct support groups. The association publishes a quarterly newsletter and pamphlets, booklets, and manuals on aspects of ostomy care and adjustment to life with an ostomy. Colostomy guides are available in English, Spanish, French, and Chinese.

Vital Options (VO), 4419 Coldwater Canyon Avenue, Suites A-C, Studio City, California 91604, (818) 508-5657, is a nonprofit organization geared to the special needs of young adults, ages 17 to 40, with cancer and other life-threatening diseases. VO offers free weekly support groups and psychotherapy sessions in California and telephone outreach counseling throughout the United States. VO publishes a newsletter entitled *Vital Times*. Descriptive materials about the organization are available from the headquarters office.

Westin Hotel Guestrooms for Cancer Patients are a cooperative effort of the ACS and the Westin Hotels. The guestrooms provide overnight accommodations for cancer patients who need them when traveling away from their homes for treatment. Many will provide for a maximum stay of six weeks per reservation, possibly longer under special circumstances. Accommodations can be provided free while patients are receiving treatment on an outpatient basis. Some Westin Hotels also accommodate family members in special instances when the patient is hospitalized. Only the ACS can make reservations for a patient, and eligibility requirements vary among the different divisions of the ACS. This program is described in a print-out from the ACS Cancer Response System.

Y-me, 18220 Harwood Avenue, Homewood, Illinois 60430, (312) 799-8338, is a not-for-profit program that provides information about breast cancer: detection and treatment; presurgical counseling and referral; educational programs; self-help meetings for breast cancer patients, their families, and friends; and, in their Homewood, Illinois, office, a wig and prosthesis bank. Their 24-hour hotline number is (312) 799-8228, and their toll-free number is (800) 221-2141. The organization publishes a newsletter and materials descriptive of its programs.

Another publication that may be helpful for your patients is the magazine *Coping: Living with Cancer*, which offers feature articles, news reports, profiles, and information on oncology research and issues for people who are living with cancer. For more information, contact Cope Publications, 377 Riverside Drive, Box 1677, Franklin, Tennessee 37065-1677, (615) 371-8474.

"Living With Cancer" is a nationally syndicated, weekly newspaper column prepared by the Norris Cotton Cancer Center in Hanover, New Hampshire, in cooperation with the New Hampshire Division of the American Cancer Society. The column answers questions from the public about cancer diagnosis, treatment, adjustment, and epidemiology. For more information, contact Columbia Features, 3500 S. Atlantic Avenue, New Smyrna Beach, Florida 32069; telephone (904) 423-2329.

Chapter 18

Rehabilitative Aspects in the Care of the Oncology Patient

With advances in early detection techniques, as well as in multimodal therapies, cancer survival rates are rising. In 1989, six million Americans who had had cancer were alive, and three million survived five years or more. After diagnosis and treatment, what is life like for these millions of cancer survivors?

Survival rates while justifiably important in themselves cover only a portion of the total problem. The rates do not relate to how the patient survives; at what cost to his physical functioning; how he adapted to his condition from a psychological point of view; and how he is fulfilling his roles, in his family, at work, among friends and in the wider society.[1]

Numerous coexisting and interrelated factors influence the quality of life of the cancer patient. Although the amount and intensity of stressors vary depending on the individual, as well as the time in the disease course, living with cancer is an on-going process that affects all domains of one's life—physical, psychological, social, and functional (see Figure 18.1).

In caring for the cancer patient, it is crucial that the various factors that affect overall well-being be addressed. With consideration and identification of the short-term and long-term effects of cancer and cancer treatment, appropriate therapeutic interventions and referrals can be employed to maximize the quality of life of the cancer patient.

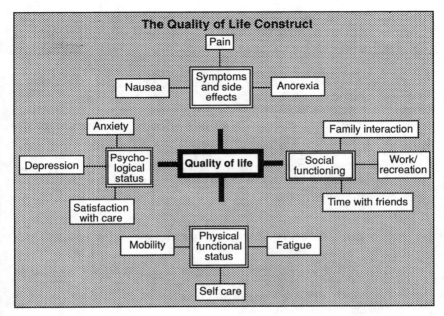

Figure 18.1. Quality of life in the cancer patient. (From -Tchekmedyian, N.S. et al., Oncology, 4, 1990, p. 186.)

SHORT-TERM EFFECTS

During the acute phase of cancer treatment, various physical symptoms and side effects may be experienced and subsequently may affect the way the cancer patient feels and functions. For example, fatigue and nausea are very common and are caused by different treatment regimens, including chemotherapy, radiation therapy, and immunotherapy. In addition to disease-related pain, pain may occur from various treatment modalities, such as chemotherapy and radiation therapy-related mucositis, or post-surgical neuritis. Due to these physical symptoms, changes in ability to participate in usual work, home, and leisure activities frequently occur.

The scheduling or frequency of treatments, hospitalizations, or outpatient appointments, as well as symptom distress, may cause the cancer patient to decrease or stop employment. The reduction in income from employment is compounded by tremendous medical bills, adding a financial burden and increased dependence to the cancer patient's list of stressors.

Among the psychosocial effects, altered body image is a common phenomenon that may result from surgery (e.g. mastectomy, orchiectomy, and colostomy), chemotherapy-induced alopecia, or changes in body weight. The physical changes frequently affect interpersonal relationships, including intimacy and sexuality. Also, these individuals may become more dependent on others for emotional support, financial aid, or assistance with activities of daily living. The myriad of physical and lifestyle changes contribute to the great challenge of coping with the diagnosis and treatment of cancer.

LONG-TERM EFFECTS

Cancer survivorship, especially in adults, is a relatively new area of study, but is highly significant. Cancer survivors could be considered those individuals who are living with persistent but controlled cancer or those who are disease-free.

In addition to chronic physical problems that may continue from cancer or cancer therapy, mental scars may exist. Lasting impressions can be characterized by easy recall of initial feelings and emotions associated with the illness and recovery period, a continuing concern about one's mortality, and an enduring sense of vulnerability.[2] Health care providers need to be sensitive to these distressing feelings of vulnerability and lack of control. Fear of recurrence has been linked to unpredictable behavior of patients, such as physician avoidance or hypochondriasis.[3] Also, while in waiting rooms for follow-up clinic appointments, this anxiety can be heightened as a result of exposure to patients with advanced cancer. It is speculated that these fears and anxieties are diminished over time.

The overall cancer experience is different for each individual and may have a positive, as well as negative, impact. Some experience increased enjoyment with each day, greater spiritual enrichment, and an increased closeness with family and friends after cancer diagnosis. Some survivors describe the diagnosis of cancer as necessary to re-evaluate priorities and make important changes in their lives.

Adjusting to the well role may be a challenge to the patient who is completing or has completed cancer therapy. Separation anxiety is a common phenomenon that occurs upon cessation of treatment. It may be manifested by an increase in outpatient visits for minor symptoms or by frequent telephone calls to health care providers.[4]

Attempting to integrate the cancer experience into the well role includes normalizing interpersonal relationships. Survivors must cope with varied responses from family, friends, and colleagues after the diagnosis of cancer. Upon treatment completion, the cancer patient may be forced to be "normal"; the intense emotional support and assistance offered during treatment may disappear when the cancer patient no longer looks or feels ill. For some individuals, it is difficult to give up the "specialness" and advantages of being sick. On the other hand, there are those family members and friends who prevent the cancer patient from resuming the usual roles and responsibilities and establishing a "normal" life. Some family members continue to react to the survivor in his or her sick role and may not be able to put the illness behind them.

Interference with intimacy and sexuality in the long-term cancer survivor may be caused by a variety of factors, including altered body image from overt physical changes, difficulty with sexual intercourse (e.g. surgically-induced impotence), or infertility (e.g. chemotherapy-induced). These factors may be exacerbated by other psychological issues, such as depression or anxiety. Andersen[5] cautions clinicians to distinguish between sexual difficulties of psychogenic origin and those physiologically related to cancer and its therapy.

Although work performance is not necessarily affected by a history of cancer, employment discrimination is an unfortunate reality for many cancer survivors. Some employers perceive cancer survivors as financially draining due to high health insurance costs or believe that they are less productive on the job. Others may view cancer as contagious or as a death sentence. Dismissal, demotion, and reduction or elimination of work-related benefits are potential work problems for the cancer survivor.[6]

Due to exorbitant health care costs, stability and comprehensiveness of health insurance are extremely important to the cancer patient. Recent studies of cancer survivors have reported a multitude of insurance barriers, including higher premiums, policy reductions or cancellations, refusal of new applications, waived or excluded pre-existing conditions, and extended waiting periods.[7] In recent years, there have been increasing federal and state laws to protect cancer patients from employment and insurance discrimination.

Physicians need to be sensitive to one of the greatest stressors of the cancer patient—the financial burden related to having cancer. It is essential to have an understanding of the various employment and insurance problems facing cancer survivors, as well as the resources and interventions that may alleviate this tremendous burden (see Chapter 16).

RESOURCES AVAILABLE WITHIN THE MEDICAL CENTER

Within most medical centers, numerous resources and services are available to assist in the comprehensive management and rehabilitation of the cancer patient. To provide the patient with the best possible care, as well as to make life easier for the house officer, it is essential to utilize the worthwhile resources listed in Table 18.1.

COMMUNITY RESOURCES AND SERVICES

Due to the trend in health care from inpatient to outpatient settings, home and community health care has been expanding. It is important to be familiar with the many valuable community resources and services available which assist cancer patients and families in coping and living with cancer at home.

Nursing services at home range from basic care to complex treatments. Visiting nurses' agencies provide care that includes dressing changes, medication monitoring, patient teaching, and reinforcement related to self-care, and assessing for possible complications. Associated with these agencies are home health aides and homemakers, that assist with activities of daily living. Meals on Wheels is a community service that delivers one nutritionally complete meal each day to one's home. Rehabilitative services are also available in the home, such as physical therapy and occupational therapy, for those that are homebound. In addition, oxygen therapy, suctioning, and inhalation treatments can be provided by home respiratory therapists.

More complex home nursing care includes home infusion therapy by highly trained and skilled registered nurses. Intravenous administration

Table 18.1
Resources Available Within the Medical Center

Behavioral Medicine	Utilize behavioral techniques such as progressive muscle relaxation, hypnosis, and imagery to assist in the management of pain, anxiety, and nausea and vomiting.
Chaplaincy	Provide pastoral counseling and emotional support to patient and families of various faiths. Offer sacraments. Consult on religious, ethical, and personal concerns.
Dietician	Consults on nutritional status and body requirements, and recommends appropriate caloric, vitamin, and mineral supplements, tube feedings, and hyperalimentation. Educates patients and families on nutritional matters, e.g., special diets or cooking hints.
Discharge Planning	Facilitates discharge process by identifying patient discharge needs, coordinating necessary home care, and initiating appropriate discharge referrals. With the implementation of DRGs and pressure to discharge patients sooner, it is increasingly important to assess discharge needs and involve a discharge planning nurse early in the patient's hospitalization.
Enterostomal Therapist	Teaches patients and families in the care and maintenance of ostomies. Consults on stomal care, skin care, and the use of appliances in patients with ostomies.
Hospice/Palliative Care Team	Consults on the care of terminally-ill patients, addressing physical, psychological, social, and spiritual needs of the dying patient and family.
Occupational Therapist	Assists with functional impairments (e.g. amputations or paralysis) to resume activities of daily living

Table 18.1
Resources Available Within the Medical Center—continued

	through the use of adaptive equipment, perceptive training, and sensory re-education.
Oncology Nurse Specialist	Consults on the care of the oncology patient including: symptom management (pain, nausea and vomiting, mucositis, bowel problems, skin care, and alopecia), chemotherapy administration and extravasation, venous access devices, research protocols, and psychosocial concerns. Provides education and counseling to cancer patients and families. Assists in the coordination of care. Participates in support groups and patient educational programs.
Pain Management Team	Multidisciplinary team (may consist of anesthesia, nursing, psychiatry, behavioral medicine, and physical therapy) which consult on the management of patients in pain.
Pharmacist	Consults on pharmacological issues such as chemotherapeutic agents, antiemetics, narcotics and other analgesics, antibiotics, and drug interactions.
Physical Therapy	Assist in the regaining and maintenance of function, endurance, and strength. Pain management through the use of hydrotherapy, as well as TENS units. Instructs breast surgery patients about exercises to improve arm and shoulder motions, and prevent lymphedema. Use fitted compression stockings and sleeves, as well as teach repositioning and exercises to minimize lymphedema. Provide chest physiotherapy to assist in the removal of pooled secretions.

Table 18.1
Resources Available Within the Medical Center—continued

Plastic Surgery	Consult on patients contemplating breast reconstruction; early consultations, prior to any breast surgery, may be beneficial to patient in decision making process. Consult on laryngectomy patients, in collaboration with otolaryngology, for voice reconstruction.
Protocol Management	Guide in the use of research protocols, including specific study directives, eligiblity criteria, and diagnostic tests. Provide information about clinical trials that are available at the institution.
Psychiatry	Consult on the clarification of affective and behavioral changes that may be difficult to decipher in the oncology patient. Guide in the use of psychotropic medications. Initiate or assist in referrals for psychotherapy.
Respiratory Therapy	Provide respiratory care, including inhalation treatments and deep suctioning. Consult on respiratory care issues, such as oxygen administration, breathing devices, and aerosol and humidity therapy.
Social Services	Assist patients and families with financial and insurance concerns. Provide information about community health and social service organizations and programs. Assist in the transfer and placement of patients to other facilities such as rehabilitative centers, nursing homes, community hospitals, and hospices. Participate in support groups and patient education programs.
Speech and Language Therapy	Assist in improving communication of patients with laryngectomies, aphasia, and dysarthria.

of antibiotics, certain types of chemotherapy, fluids, hyperalimentation, and narcotics are possible in the home setting for patients and families that are motivated and capable. It is easier to provide these treatments with an indwelling venous device (port or catheter), although many of the advanced technological home nursing agencies are able to provide peripheral venous access if necessary.

Insurance coverage for the many home care and nursing services varies, depending on the company and policy. In general, at least a portion of the services are covered for appropriate patients. It is surmised that insurance coverage will expand for these services along with the trend in outpatient health care.

Hospice is a coordinated interdisciplinary program of supportive services and pain and symptom control for terminally-ill patients and their families. Hospice programs differ in scope of care, structure, and organization; they range from grassroots interest groups that rely heavily on professional and lay volunteers to organizations that provide comprehensive palliative and support services through employees and lay volunteers. Most programs provide home care services and support that assist individuals in dying at home if they choose to. In addition to home hospice care there are a limited number of freestanding hospices throughout the country which are facilities that solely provide holistic inpatient care to terminally-ill patients and families.

Most medical centers and communities have a variety of support groups for patients and families. Support groups assist individuals in similar situations to cope with their medical condition or life stressors. The populations and focus for the groups may vary: type of disease (e.g. cancer in general, lung cancer, and breast cancer); type of surgery (e.g. laryngectomy, ostomy, and mastectomy); and family (caregivers, bereavement, and spouses). Most support groups affiliated with medical centers are facilitated by professionals who are usually nurses, social workers, or chaplains.

REFERENCES

1. Izsack, F.C., and Medalie, J.H. (1971). Comprehensive follow-up of carcinoma patients. *Journal of Chronic Diseases*, 24:179–191.
2. Shanfield, S.B. (1980). On surviving cancer: psychological considerations. *Comprehensive Psychiatry*, 21:128–134.

3. Mullan, F. (1984). Re-entry: the educational needs of the cancer survivor. *Health Education Quarterly*, 10 (supp.):88–94.
4. Gorzynski, J.G., and Holland, J.C. (1979). Psychological aspects of testicular cancer. *Seminars in Oncology*, 6:125–129.
5. Andersen, B. L. (1985). Sexual functioning morbidity among cancer survivors. *Cancer*, 55:1935–42.
6. Welch-McCaffrey, D., Hoffman, B., Leigh, S., Loescher, L. J., and Meyskens, F.L. (1989). Surviving adult cancers. Part 2: Psychosocial implications. *Annals of Internal Medicine*, 111:517–524.
7. Crothers, H. (1987). Health insurance: problems and solutions for people with cancer histories. In: *Proceedings of the Fifth National Conference on Human Values and Cancer*. San Francisco: American Cancer Society, 100–109.

Chapter 19

Important Points about Specific Cancers

The cancers discussed in this chapter are listed in alphabetical order. Specific information on any cancer updated monthly can be obtained easily through CancerFax at 1-301-402-5874.

BLADDER CANCER

1. There is a new excitement about the treatment of bladder cancer with recently discovered effective combination chemotherapy regimens like "M-VAC" and "CMV," described below.

2. Bladder cancer is seen more frequently in males (felt to be due in part to occupational exposure). Cancers are often multicentric (called a "field change" by exposure of the urothelium to carcinogens).

3. Papillomas develop into invasive disease in 7% of cases. There is a 30% chance of developing a second papilloma if you have had one; there is a 70% chance if you have had two.

   In situ cancers (called TIS) are often multicentric and in 32–83% of cases, invasive cancers develop in patients with TIS lesions.

   Flow cytometry of urine cytology provides clues to future invasiveness (cells with >16% DNA index or aneuploidy are more likely to progress).

4. Staging

	Marshall/ Jewett-Strong	TNM
No tumor-definitive specimen		T_0
Carcinoma in situ	0	T_{IS}
Papillary tumor without invasion	0	T_a
Invasion lamina propria	A	T_1
Superficial muscle invasion	B_1	T_2
Deep muscle invasion	B_2	$T3_a$
Invasion perivesical fat	C	$T3_b$
Invasion contiguous viscera	D_1	$T4_a$
Pelvic nodes	D_1	N_{1-3}
Nodes above aortic bifurcation	D_2	N_4
Distant metastases	D_2	M

5. Superficial disease—stages T_a and T_1 (90% of cancers)—has increased in incidence. This is treated by TURB (transurethral resection). Intravesical chemotherapy decreases recurrences and subsequent development of invasive cancers. Agents used include BCG, thiotepa, mitomycin-C and Adriamycin. If intravesical therapy doesn't control recurrences, or if diffuse multifocal TIS is present or recurs, a cystectomy should be performed.

6. Muscle invasive disease. Options for treatment include: cystectomy only, pre-op or post-op radiation plus cystectomy, chemotherapy plus cystectomy, or radiation alone with salvage cystectomy if necessary.

The NCI has a group of protocols called "high priority" trials. The questions these ask are most important for cancer care in the United States. One of the most interesting asks the question if chemotherapy (M-VAC) prior to cystectomy is better than cystectomy alone. Early results look favorable for the combination.

The following excerpt shows how these high priority trials are advertised to patients:

What is the Purpose of the Study?

The National Cancer Institute (NCI) is sponsoring a study of bladder cancer treatments that could lead to increased survival for many bladder cancer patients.

This study compares one of the standard treatments for bladder cancer—surgical removal of the bladder, called cystectomy—to 4-drug combination chemotherapy (anticancer drugs) followed by surgery. Standard treatments for bladder cancer often prolong patient survival but fail to cure the majority of patients with more advanced bladder cancer. Researchers have reason to believe that chemotherapy given before surgery may increase survival and lessen the chances of tumor recurrence. In initial studies, chemotherapy appeared very effective in bladder cancer patients. Seventy percent of chemotherapy patients responded favorably, with the tumor shrinking; in a third of these responding patients, the tumor disappeared.

7. Cystectomy alone, pre-op (low dose) radiation with cystectomy, and high dose radiation with salvage cystectomy produce about the same results. Another trial to be done will study chemotherapy followed by high dose radiation with the goal of bladder preservation.

8. CMV (cisplatinum, methotrexate, velban) and M-VAC (the same drugs plus Adriamycin) appear to be the most active regimens, reporting 50–60% response rates (complete plus partial remissions).

   Studies are in progress using these regimens as adjuvant therapy, as well as pre-surgery (neoadjuvant) as described above.

9. Summary (see Fig. 19.1)

BREAST CANCER

1. Approximately 130,000 cases of breast cancer occur annually in U.S. There is a 10% lifetime risk for an American woman (about 7% before age 70) and the incidence is rising.

2. Breast cancer usually (90%) presents with a painless lump discovered accidentally or by self-examination. Occasionally breast carcinomas are painful, however. Inflammatory changes, dimpling of skin (due to underlying traction), nipple distortion, and bloody discharge may also occur.

3. Any suspicious breast mass should be considered for mammography. At times a true carcinoma is found nearby when the original mass noted is benign. The false negative rate of mammography is about 5–10% dependent on density of breast tissue, location of tumor (e.g. just

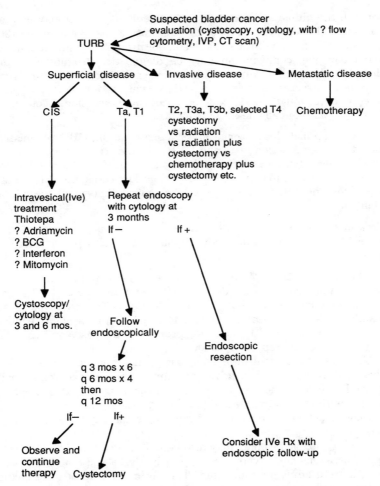

Figure 19.1

beneath the nipple is difficult to see). Needle aspiration may help determine if the lesion is cystic or demonstrate a positive cytology (90% accuracy). For a small tumor, a needle localization in conjunction with mammographic confirmation may be diagnostic. Prognostic studies should be done whenever possible on biopsied material; these include estrogen/progesterone receptors, DNA analysis for ploidy, S phase fraction determination, HER-2/neu oncogene expression. (You should find out what is available at your institution.)

4. The work up includes history, physical examination, CBC, chemistries including liver function tests and CXR. A bone scan may be done as a baseline, or if lymph node involvement is suspected clinically but less than 3% are found to be positive with stage I or II disease. Liver scans are of low yield in the absence of biochemical abnormalities or hepatomegaly.

5. Treatment will be discussed by stage.
   Stages I and II (i.e. those with small tumors and positive axillary nodes).

   The treatments of choice seem to be modified radical mastectomy versus some form of local excision combined with radiation. The more extensive surgeries are not currently being performed as often and results are similar no matter which form of local treatment. Axillary node dissection should be done for prognostic purposes and to determine if further therapy is needed.

   The addition of adjuvant chemotherapy has produced a median survival and overall survival advantage for premenopausal women with stage II cancer. The results are also promising for premenopausal women with stage I cancer and poor prognostic signs (i.e. unfavorable histology, lack of estrogen receptor proteins and expression of certain oncogenes).

   Postmenopausal women may also benefit from adjuvant chemotherapy. Postmenopausal women with positive ER's and stage II disease benefit from adjuvant tamoxifen. The optimal duration of tamoxifen therapy is yet to be defined.

Locally advanced breast cancer

This group includes patients who may be unresectable technically, inoperable or those with inflammatory changes. They may not have distant metastases but local disease control by surgery alone has proven to be unlikely.

These patients are now given chemotherapy first. If they have a complete clinical response, radiation alone or with a mastectomy is then given. If a partial response occurs, radiation is then used. If the tumor is resectable, surgery is done. If not resectable, more chemotherapy is given.

Metastatic disease

Numerous options are available from surgical excision of local recurrence to local radiation for symptomatic metastases. Systemic treatment options depend on site(s) of metastasis, disease duration and disease free interval, estrogen and progesterone receptor status, age, prior treatment results (see Table 19.1).

6. Estrogen receptor levels help in the selection of therapy. Those patients with high levels or simultaneously positive progesterone receptors are more likely to respond. (One should also consider hormonal therapy in those patients with progesterone receptors only since the lack of estrogen receptors may be an artifact in such patients.)

In general, the sequence of hormonal choices in a premenopausal woman is as follows: a) oophorectomy or tamoxifen, b) whichever of those two that wasn't chosen first, c) progestationals, d) aminoglutethamide, e) androgens or glucocorticoids.

The sequence in a postmenopausal woman is: a) tamoxifen; b) progestationals; c) aminoglutethamide; d) androgens or glucocorticoids.

7. Reconstructive surgery is becoming highly developed with excellent cosmetic results.

CENTRAL NERVOUS SYSTEM TUMORS

1. There are 12,000 new cases of primary CNS tumors per year. CNS tumors are the second most common cancer in children.

2. CNS tumors can be divided into those arising from neuroectodemal origin and those arising from mesodermal origin (e.g. meningiomas). The neuroectodermal tumors can be divided into the "relatively benign" astrocytomas and oligodendrogliomas and the more malignant anaplastic astrocytoma and glioblastoma multiforme. Gliomas are divided by grade into a) astrocytomas, b) anaplastic astrocytomas (with

Table 19.1
Principles of Systemic Treatment of Metastatic Breast Cancer

1. Attempt to control the disease process and associated symptoms with as gentle a treatment as can reasonably be effective (e.g. hormonal therapy in older women). The gentlest therapies appear to be tamoxifen or megare.
2. Reserve more debilitating regimens (palliative intent) for the time when they become necessary to relieve symptoms.
3. One hormonal response suggests that other hormonal response may occur sequentially with different agents (or by simply stopping an ineffective but previously successful regimen).
4. A postmenopausal woman with positive or unknown receptors, or a long disease free interval, or with modest organ involvement is a candidate for hormonal treatment. Two consecutive unsuccessful hormonal trials is strongly usggestive of hormone refractoriness.
5. A patient with aggressive visceral involvement (liver, lung, widely destructive bone lesions) usually merits chemotherappy, unless receptors are definitely high. Numerous potentially effective chemoterapy agents are available with doxorubicin regarded as the most active and combinations of cyclophosphamide, 5-FU, and doxorubicin or methotrexate most commonly used.
6. A beneficial hormone response may take as long as two months to see, and ocasionally a response to chemotherapy is not seen until 3–6 months after beginning treatment.
7. For selected younger patients with metastatic (or very likely metastatic) disease who exhibit a good response to chemotherapy, bone marrow transplantation is an investigational option potentially capable of achieving long term control.

increased cellular pleomorphism and vascular hyperplasia) and c) glioblastoma multiforme.

3. Since they occur in an enclosed space, all expanding masses within the CNS can cause death. In contrast to systemic cancer in which 1 gram of tumor is lethal, within the CNS 100 mg of tumor plus surrounding edema can be lethal.

4. CNS tumors do not metastasize but cause death by expanding locally. The more malignant tumors grow more rapidly and infiltrate more widely.

5. CNS tumors present with either generalized or focal neurological signs. The CT scan is the most useful diagnostic test. The MRI is more sensitive, expecially for low grade and posterior fossa tumors.

6. Diagnosis can be confirmed either by stereotaxic or open biopsy.

7. Surgery is the usual first treatment. Cytoreduction by debulking (if complete resection is impossible) may ameliorate symptoms and improve the effectiveness of radiation.

8. Radiation is the therapy utilized the most. The usual dose is 6000 rads with a focal boost for malignant tumors and 5000–5500 rads for astrocytomas.

9. New strategies in radiation include:
   a. the use of radiosensitizers (theoretically important but practically not much improvement to date)
   b. different fractionation schemes (e.g. twice a day)
   c. use of neutrons or other particles
   d. implantation of radioactive seeds
   e. hyperthermia

10. There are not many "effective" chemotherapeutic agents. The "best" appears to be BCNU, and this combined with RT gives a marginal survival benefit. One problem for delivery of effective drugs is the "blood-brain" barrier. More drug gets into the tumor than into the brain, though.

11. One of the best ways to improve symptoms is effective use of corticosteroids. Decadron 4 mg, q6h is the usual dose.

12. Anticonvulsants should be used if seizures have occurred.

13. Median survival time even using the most "effective" therapy is 1 year with about 30% of patients alive at 18 months.

14. CNS lymphomas are being seen more commonly in patients with AIDS and other immunodeficiency states. These have been linked to Epstein-Barr virus.

15. Remember rehabilitation and consult the electronic databases for the latest information (see Chapter 20 for new developments).

CERVICAL CANCER

1. There are 13,000 cases annually in US, with the peak incidence between ages 48–55. Generally carcinoma is preceded by dysplasia and carcinoma in situ. Women with AIDS may have rapidly progressive, multicentric and recurrent cervical cancer.

2. Usually the disease is assymptomatic but with invasion discharge or bleeding may occur. Pain, rectal or urinary tract symptoms generally occur late in course of disease.

3. The staging workup generally includes CXR, cystoscopy, sigmoidoscopy, IVP, barium enema, and CT scan to assess nodal architecture.

4. With a frankly abnormal Pap smear, colposcopy and/or biopsy is done. For dysplasias and in situ lesions (CIN 1–3), cryotherapy, laser therapy or cone biopsy may be done. Also, hysterectomy may be performed. For invasive cancer, radical hysterectomy (Total abdominal hysterectomy and bilateral salpingo-oophorectomy) or radiation to the pelvis with intraca vitary therary is performed. If the disease extends locally out of the cervix, radiation is used preoperatively. A key to prognosis is assessment of the paraaortic nodes. If positive, radiation to the nodes and the pelvis is done. In addition, chemotherapy has also been used. If the nodes are negative, pelvic radiation plus intracavitary implants are used.

5. Chemotherapeutic agents of moderate value in metastatic or advanced disease include cisplatinum, ifosfamide, 5FU, vincristine, cyclophosphamide. Platinum is also being used as a radiation sensitizer in combined modality treatments.

COLON, RECTAL, AND ANAL CANCER

1. Overall, cancers of the colon and rectum are the second most common cancer in the U.S. Colon cancer accounts for approximately 44,000 cases, with equal numbers occurring in both sexes. There has been a trend toward more cases developing in the proximal colon. There has also been a gradual improvement in the survival rate over the past quarter century, and this probably is not related to better therapy.

2. A change in bowel habits is often the first symptom and may be very non-specific, depending on the tumor location. Iron deficiency anemia is often the first sign of the disease, particularly in proximal bowel lesions. In distal lesions, frank blood in the stool may be seen, along with symptoms of rectal urgency or tenesmus. Some patients will present with symptoms of bowel obstruction.

3. Careful history and physical examination along with digital rectal examination and stool for occult blood should be performed. Rigid or preferably flexible sigmoidoscopy or colonoscopy should be performed, at which time a biopsy may be obtained. Barium studies with or without air contrast may be very helpful in establishing the diagnosis. Routine laboratory studies including a CBC and liver function studies will be helpful.

4. There are several histologic types, the most important being adenocarcinoma with varying degrees of differentiation. In the anal canal, there are several different cell types with different biologic behaviors, including squamous carcinomas and carcinomas of the transitional epithelium (cloacogenic carcinomas).

5. Once the diagnosis of colorectal carcinoma is made much of the actual staging occurs intraoperatively. Liver function studies should be performed and if abnormal should be followed by a liver imaging procedure such as a CT scan or ultrasound. Nevertheless, in most cases the patient will need exploration for removal or bypass of the obstructing lesion. Staging is based on local-regional and distant disease spread using the Duke's staging system, based on degree of penetration through the intestinal wall, regional lymph node involvement, and spread to other organs.

6. Surgery is the primary treatment for colorectal cancer with resection of the segment of the involved intestine and reanastomosis. In low rectal lesions, an abdominal-perineal resection may be necessary. Newer sphincter sparing procedures are being investigated. Pre- or postoperative radiation therapy is beneficial in preventing local recurrences in rectal carcinoma. The exact role of radiation plus chemotherapy as an adjuvant for rectal cancer is undergoing intensive clinical trials but it appears very promising.

   Chemotherapy also may help improve the survival when given as an adjuvant in colon cancer. Recently, the combination of 5 fluorouracil and levamisole (an antiparasite drug) has been known to be effective in the adjuvant setting in patients with Duke's stage C colon cancer. The death rate has been reduced 33%.

7. Treatment for metastatic disease remains poor. 5-Fluorouracil, given via a number of schedules, has been the mainstay of chemotherapy for the past 45 years with an objective response rate of 10–20%. Recently it has been shown that when combined with leucovorin (which shunts the 5-FU into another metabolic pathway) an improved response rate (30–40%) can be obtained. This increased response rate is also accompanied by an increased toxicity.

8. Multiple chemoprevention trials are ongoing to ascertain if certain additives to the diet (e.g. vitamins A, C, E, calcium) can decrease the development of cancers in patients at high risk (i.e. those with known colonic polyps).

9. CEA (carcinoembryonic antigen) levels are often elevated in patients with colon cancer. However, this test is too non-specific and insensitive to be used in a screening situation, but can be used for followup of disease after primary (surgical) therapy. Some surgeons find a rising CEA an early indication for a repeat laparotomy to attempt to resect recurrent disease. This is especially successful if the recurrence is only at the surgical anastomosis.

10. There is increasing interest in hepatic resections of the liver involved with single metastases or those localized to one lobe.

11. Infusion pumps for intrahepatic infusion or continuous infusion of 5-FU and other agents have been utilized, but trials show only marginal differences (if any) in survival.

12. Anal cancer seems to respond well to radiation and 5-fluorouracil plus mitomycin chemotherapy.

ENDOMETRIAL CANCER

1. There are 34,000 cases annually in U.S., but fortunately, 80% are confined to uterus. It is seen especially in 55–60 year old group and risk factors include exogeneous estrogen use, nulliparity, obesity, late menopause, hypertension and diabetes mellitus.

2. Abnormal vaginal bleeding is the usual presenting symptom. Pain is suggestive of advanced disease. The diagnosis is made from cellular material provided by fractional dilation and curettage.

3. The workup includes pelvic exam, CXR, IVP, barium enema, cystoscopy, sigmoidoscopy, and CT scan of pelvis. Grade is also an important prognostic factor.

4. Stage I endometrial cancer is confined to the endometrium and hysterectomy and bilateral salpingo-oophorectomy is the treatment of choice. If there is deep myometrial invasion or the tumor is poorly differentiated (grade 3), post operative radiation therapy is added. For tumors invading the cervix, pre-op whole pelvis radiation is added with an intracavitary application of cesium preceding a TAH-BSO. For advanced local disease, external radiation with brachytherapy application is utilized.

5. Progestational agents (e.g. megestrol) have moderate activity against well-differentiated tumors. Response correlates with the level of progesterone receptors. Doxorubicin, platinum, and hexamethylmelamine are the most active chemotherapeutic agents.

ESOPHAGEAL CANCER

1. Esophageal carcinoma accounts for approximately 10,000 cases per year. The geographical distribution of this neoplasm varies widely throughout the world with the highest rates being seen in China. A number of putative causative relationships with dietary constituents, and especially smoking and alcohol have been found. There may be a shift in the type of this cancer in the United States with more adenocarcinomas being discovered in the past decade. (More than 50% of adenocarcinomas of the esophagus are associated with Barrett's esophagus.) The etiologic factors for these are probably different.

2. Screening is done in high prevalence areas in China by a "Lawary"—an inflatable balloon covered by nylon or silk mesh pulled through the esophagus. The specimens obtained are examined cytologically. Some in the U.S. favor screening esophago-gastroscopy in patients with Barrett's.

3. Dysphagia is the primary symptom of both types of carcinoma. This is associated with weight loss, and sometimes with pain radiating to

back. Other symptoms are generally due to metastatic disease. Occasionally tracheo-esophageal fistulae occur.

4. Biopsy via endoscope is necessary. Most patients have a barium swal-
low prior to this. CT scans of the chest are helpful in staging and should
include the liver and upper retroperitoneum. Routine chest x-ray and
lab studies should be performed.

5. Squamous carcinomas generally spread locally or regionally, and distant metastatic sites usually occur late in the course. Since the esophagus contains no serosa, local extension is common and, because of the
rich lymphatics in the submucosa, wide dissemination along the esophagus is common.

6. Surgical resection is the primary treatment modality for cure. Radiation therapy may cure a small fraction of patients. In some series tri-
modality therapy using chemotherapy, radiation and surgery has led
to improved "cure" rates in very selected patients. The primary treatment for most patients is palliative and consists of treatments to maintain swallowing function and nutrition for as long as possible.

7. Chemotherapy, especially with carboplatinum, may induce responses,
and the use of chemotherapy in combined modality programs is actively being explored.

8. Palliation of dysplagia with intraesophageal tubes or laser therapy may
also be utilized. Laser therapy, although effective in 60–70% of patients, usually needs to be repeated every 6 to 8 weeks.

9. Survival in this disease is poor, with only about 5% of patients surviving 5 years.

HEAD AND NECK CANCER

1. There are approximately 42,000 cases per year in the U.S., with a
male to female ratio of 3:1. H and N cancer includes all carcinomas
arising in squamous mucosal epithelium from the lip, oral and nasal
cavities, pharynx to the larynx. They all have a common etiology (cigarette smoking and alcohol seem to be additive risk factors; smokeless
tobacco, pipe smoking, and marijuana smoking also appear to carry
increased risk). In Canton (China) EB virus is associated with nasopharyngeal carcinoma.

2. All smokers (especially those who also abuse alcohol) should have a careful exam of the oral cavity. Early lesions may show only surface erythema and roughened mucosa. A mass or ulcerated area may be noted, or hoarseness, neck nodes, pain radiating to the ear, or nasal congestion may be chief complaints. The complaint of hoarseness should stimulate an exam of the larynx. The vocal cords are devoid of lymphatics, tumors tend to stay localized there for longer periods and hoarseness occurs early in the course.

3. If a suspicious neck node is encountered, a careful search for a head and neck primary is paramount (ENT consultation)—"blind" biopsies are appropriate if a primary lesion is not found. For any patient, there should be a complete assessment of other potential sites for second primaries (e.g. esophagus and tracheobronchial tree).

4. The work-up includes complete history and physical examination, CBC and chemistry profile, CXR, CT scan of involved area, and "triple" endoscopy. The staging format is dependent on the particular primary site in TNM system and is different from area to area within the H and N. It will not be reproduced here. The tumor spreads generally at first to local node groups. Unless lymphoma or arising from the salivary glands, squamous cell histology is almost universal.

5. For H and N cancer, a multidisciplinary approach is now favored with surgery and/or radiation therapy for local eradication of disease. For early stage lesions either surgery or radiation therapy may suffice. Radiation therapy is the primary treatment for tumors arising in the nasopharynx. Combination chemotherapy (e.g. platinum and 5-FU are often given prior to local treatment, since response rates are quite high (75%) and systemic treatment may eradicate early metastases. Even with complete remission of the tumor, surgical and radiation therapy principles related to the extent of local treatment remain the same (i.e. if the extent of tumor was deemed worthy of radical; dissection at outset, even with a complete remission on chemotherapy, the same surgery is performed). Salvage laryngectomy may be performed if recurrence occurs after radiation.

6. Chemotherapy for recurrent carcinomas is palliative—weekly methotrexate is a reasonable choice. Platinum and 5-FU are also useful agents. Advanced disease may be complicated by hypercalcemia, malnutrition and fistulae.

7. Reconstructive surgery can add to functional and cosmetic aspects. Remember to refer patients to physical therapy and for voice rehabilitation if necessary.

8. Surveillance for second tumors is very important in these patients.

KAPOSI'S SARCOMA

1. In the past, Kaposi's sarcoma (KS) was mosy commonly seen in the Mediterranean area and was characterized by "idiopathic, multiple pigmented sarcomas of skin." It was also seen in patients with kidney transplants, but now is most commonly seen in patients with immunodeficiency diseases, especially AIDS. In AIDS, the tumor has a tendency to appear in the oral cavity and anal area.

2. It most often presents with multiple red cutaneous macules which may ulcerate, but generally are not symptomatic. Dyspnea and hemoptysis may be seen with pulmonary lesions.

3. It also may present with lymphadenopathy providing a source for tissue. The diagnosis is usually made by cutaneous biopsy.

4. Staging
   - Stage I = cutaneous, locally indolent.
   - Stage II = cutaneous, locally aggressive with or without regional node involvement.
   - Stage III = generalized mucocutaneous or lymph node involvement, or both.
   - Stage IV = visceral involvement
                Subtype A = no systemic signs or symptoms.
                Subtype B = systemic signs such as weight loss, fever.
                ("B" symptoms are associated with a poorer prognosis.)
   The workup includes physical exam, CBC, CXR, serum chemistries, and appropriate additional studies determined by symptoms and signs.

5. Treatment
   Interferons have objective response rates of 25–40%—no benefit is seen when vinblastine or VP-16 is added.
   Vinblastine, VP-16 and Adriamycin have moderate activity as single agents.
   KS lesions are radiosensitive.

KIDNEY CANCER

1. Renal carcinoma or "hypernephroma" accounts for approximately 23,000 new cases per year. Because of its propensity to present with a variety of syndromes, such as fever, hypercalcemia, or hepatic dysfunction in the absence of direct liver invasion, it has also been called the "internists' tumor." Like melanoma, its behavior is often different than other cancers, and it can have periods of long stability followed by explosive disease. It is also one of the diseases where some of the newer biologic therapy may be of benefit. In some cases, surgical resection of metastases may be beneficial.

2. The "classic" triad of painless hematuria, abdominal mass and pain occurs in only 20% of patients. One or more of these symptoms is seen in well over 60% of cases. Other symptoms are listed below:

Symptom	Incidence (%)
Elevated E.S.R.	55.6
Anemia	41.3
Hypertension	37.6
Fever	34.5
Abnormal liver function tests	15.0
Elevated alkaline phosphatase	14.7
Hypercalcemia	5.7
Polycythemia	3.7
Neuromyopathy	3.3
Amyloidosis	2.1

3. Radiologic techniques including IVPs, kidney ultrasound, computed tomography, or renal arteriography can suggest with a high degree of certainty the diagnosis of kidney carcinoma. The findings are so characteristic that a biopsy prior to definitive surgical removal is often not warranted (Fig 19.2).

4. Surgery is the only method for cure and in many cases for staging. Pre- or postoperative radiation therapy has not been shown to be of benefit. Control of local symptoms or of associated syndromes should be considered even in patients with metastatic disease (e.g. a nephrectomy may be indicated if refractory bleeding, hypercalcemia or pain).

5. Removal of single site metastases should be considered for "cure" in selected patients (necrosis in the lesion is associated with a good prog-

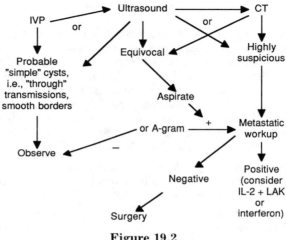

Figure 19.2

nosis) It is generally radioresistant but some palliation of pain can often be achieved with bone metastases. This tumor is equally chemotherapy resistant, although vinlastine has activity at the 5-10% level. Interleukin 2 plus LAK cells may cause regression in as many as 20% of patients. Alpha-interferon also has activity in 10–20%.

LEUKEMIAS: ACUTE MYELOID LEUKEMIA (AML) AND ACUTE LYMPHOCYTIC LEUKEMIA (ALL)

1. In adults, there are approximately 6300 new cases of AML per year and 900 new cases of ALL per year (ALL is much more common in childhood). The incidence of AML increases steadily with age, whereas with adult ALL, there is a fairly constant rate until age 65, after which it increases. Males are affected slightly more commonly than females. Unfortunately, in adults the mortality rates for the acute leukemias are about 80% of the incidence rates per year.

2. Patients with AML or ALL may present with symptoms of fatigue (due to anemia), bleeding (due to thrombocytopenia and/or DIC), or infection (due to granulocytopenia). Those with AML may have gin-

gival hypertrophy (monocytic M5 or myelomonocytic subtypes M4) or DIC (promyelocytic subtype-M3). Patients with ALL may have lymphadenopathy or splenomegaly. 15% of adults with ALL will present with, or later develop, meningeal leukemia presenting with headaches and/or cranial nerve findings. Only 5% of patients with AML will have this complication.

3. The diagnosis is usually made by looking at the CBC with differential and platelet count. A bone marrow aspiration and biopsy will provide the definitive diagnosis showing increased numbers of blasts (<5% is normal). Special histochemistry stains and phenotyping with monoclonal antibodies may differentiate AML from ALL, and help subclassify the subtypes. Occasionally, all studies will be negative and a patient will carry the diagnosis of undifferentiated leukemia.

4. AML has seven subtypes defined by the French-American-British (FAB) classification system:

    M1 Cells undifferentiated, with occasional granules.

    M2 Blasts with some maturation to promyelocyte.

    M3 Acute promyelocytic leukemia. Promyelocytes predominate.

    M4 Acute myelomonocytic leukemia. Both myeloid and monocytic-type cells present. Serum lysozyme elevated.

    M5 Acute monocytic leukemia. Monoblasts and monocytic precursors are predominant cells present.

    M6 Erythroleukemia. Megaloblastoid red cell precursors are predominant cells present.

    M7 Megakaryocytic leukemia. Cells usually phenotypically identified as megakaryocytic in origin.

    ALL has three FAB subtypes:

    L1 Small blasts with scant cytoplasm and usually one nucleolus.

    L2 More variable size and shape of cells which are usually larger than L1. Irregular nucleus with multiple nucleoli.

    L3 Large cells with basophilic cytoplasm and vacuoles may be present. Nucleus round with multiple nucleoli.

5. Most ALL is of pre-B cell phenotype. Those patients with T cell ALL often have a mediastinal mass. This occurs more frequently in males, and has a very bad prognosis. True B-cell ALL has an even worse prognosis.

6. Standard therapy for AML involves induction chemotherapy (the classic regimen is 7 days of cytosine arabinoside, or Ara-C, and 3 days

of daunorubicin) and is aimed at attaining a complete remission (CR). Older patients with multiple underlying medical problems may elect less vigorous therapy with single oral agents such as 6-mercaptopurine, or mild combination chemotherapy with agents such as cyclophosphamide, vincristine, cytosine arabinoside and prednisone. Once a complete remission is achieved, patients usually receive some form of consolidation and/or intensification therapy for 1–4 cycles followed by a maintenance phase of therapy for a short period of time. The need for maintenance therapy after repeated cycles of intensive therapy (intensification or consolidation) in AML is unclear. Patients may elect to have their own bone marrow harvested and stored for future use in an autologous bone marrow transplant. Younger patients (age <45) with an HLA-matched sibling may proceed with an allogeneic transpl ant in first remission.

7. ALL is treated initially with induction chemotherapy with a vincris tine and prednisone-based regimen. L-asparaginase and daunorubicin are other agents commonly used. Once a CR is achieved patients will often undergo repeated intensive consolidation courses of chemotherapy including agents such as Ara-C, methotrexate, VP-16, and 6-mercaptopurine. Intrathecal methotrexate and whole brain radiation are given as prophylaxis against meningeal leukemia.

8. 50–80% of patients with AML will achieve a CR with aggressive induction chemotherapy. With the oral single agent treatment only 15% will achieve a CR. With milder combination therapy about 15–40% may achieve CR status. Once CR is achieved, 15–35% of patients will remain disease free greater than two years. More recent intensive consolidation programs may improve this to 40% at best. Autologous bone marrow transplantation in first CR may yield a disease-free survival (DFS) at two years as high as 50%. Similarly, allogeneic HLA-matched transplants have a 45–60% two year DFS.

9. With relapse in AML, cure is infrequent without some form of bone marrow transplantation. Autologous and allogeneic transplantation have two year survivals of 25–30%. There is a higher relapse rate with autologous transplantation, and with allogeneic transplantation, there is higher mortality due to graft-versus-host-disease (GVHD) and interstitial pneumonitis.

10. There is a high remission rate (60–90%) for patients with adult ALL; however, long term survival has been poor. In recent studies up to

30% of patients who achieve complete remission may survive 4 years. Those with poor prognostic features at diagnosis (high WBC, CNS disease, B-cell disease, Philadelphia chromosome positivity) may consider a bone marrow transplant in first remission. As with AML, once relapse occurs, long term survival is rare in the absence of a bone marrow transplant.

LEUKEMIAS: CHRONIC MYELOGENOUS LEUKEMIA (CML), CHRONIC LYMPHOCYTIC LEUKEMIA (CLL), AND HAIRY CELL LEUKEMIA (HCL)

1. The incidence of CML is highest in the fourth to fifth decades of life, and is very rare in the first ten years of life. (Children may get a form of CML called juvenile CML, which is a different disease entity and will not be covered further here.)

2. CLL has a higher incidence than the other leukemias and most patient s are older. The median age at diagnosis is in the seventh decade, and the incidence continues to rise through the 90's. In fact, in those people 80–84 years old the incidence is 30.4 per 100,000 per year.

3. Most patients with CML will be asymptomatic at the time of diagnosis. Those with symptoms will complain of fatigue, weight loss, low grade fevers and/or night sweats. Occasionally patients may have symptoms associated with splenomegaly. With very high white counts, leukostasis may occur. The physical exam may be normal, or there may be mild to moderate splenomegaly. The presence of chloromas (extramedullary collections of leukemic cells) is a poor prognostic sign.

4. CLL may also be asymptomatic at diagnosis with the only abnormality being a lymphocytosis which may remain stable for years. As the disease progresses, lymphadenopathy develops, and later enlargement of the spleen and/or liver. Fatigue is a prominent early complaint, often in the absence of an anemia. Some patients may develop recurrent infections in association with hypogammaglobulinemia, which usually accompanies the disease. Complications associated with thrombocytopenia occur late in the course.

5. The classic presentation of HCL is pancytopenia and splenomegaly. Circulating abnormal lymphocytes are evident, that may have hair-

like projections. Patients with HCL are prone to infections with bacteria or opportunistic organisms (especially atypical mycobacteria). They may also develop autoimmune or connective tissue diseases, such as vasculitis in up to 30% of cases. Patients with HCL usually don't have enlarged nodes, and monocytes are absent from the peripheral smear.

6. The CBC with differential white blood cell count is the key to diagnosis in these diseases. Bone marrow studies will help confirm. Patients with CML will have high WBC's with all forms of myeloid cells often present as well as increased numbers of eosinophils and basophils. Platelet counts are usually high. Leukocyte alkaline phosphatase (LAP) activity is low, in contrast to patients with a reactive leukocytosis where the LAP is usually high. Cytogenetics are important to do on the marrow since at least 90% of patients will have a marker called the Philadelphia (Ph1) chromosome, usually t(9,22). Other tests often elevated are vitamin B12 and B12 binding proteins. The following table helps discriminate CML from a "leukemoid" reaction:

Reaction	CML	"Leukemoid"
Eosinophils Basophils	Present	Usually not present
LAP	Low	Normal
B12 (B12 binding)	High	Normal
Chromosomes	Ph1 present in most cases	Normal

7. CLL patients have a lymphocytosis of greater than 15,000 at diagnosis. The cells are usually mature lymphs, and phenotyping will confirm the clonal nature of these cells (usually B cell, with kappa or lambda light chain on the surface). A few patients can have a T-cell origin. The T cells are more likely to be large granular lymphs and the patients with this are more likely to have prior rheumatologic disorders. Most patients have low gamma globulin levels, and there is an increased incidence of autoimmune hemolytic anemia and/or thrombocytopenia in B-cell CLL.

As noted, patients with HCL have pancytopenia at presentation and usually their marrow is not aspirable ("dry tap"). Biopsies will show increased reticulin and diffuse infiltration with abnormal lymphs. Diagnosis is usually based on the TRAP stain (the cells show resistance to tartrate on acid phosphatase stain, unlike other lymphocytes).

8. CML is a clonal disorder at the level of the multipotential stem cell. Studies have shown that the red cells, platelets, myeloid cells, monocytes, and some populations of lymphocytes are involved. Marrow fibroblasts are not. When marrow fibrosis develops, as it often does, the fibroblasts are not derived from the malignant clone. In most cases, marrow biopsies will show marked hypercellularity with a predominance of myeloid precursors.

   The marrow cellularity in CLL will be increased due to a diffuse infiltration with mature lymphocytes. A rarer entity, prolymphocytic leukemia, will show larger, more immature lymphoid cells with prominent nucleoli.

9. CML has three phases. The chronic phase (CP) is usually present at diagnosis, and patients usually have few symptoms with elevation of the white blood count the predominant finding. Over time, patients will often evolve to an accelerated phase (AP), which is intermediate between the chronic phase and the terminal phase, also called blast crisis (BC). The transition to AP is gradual over one or more months. More difficulty controlling the WBC, high platelet counts (> 1 million/mm^3), increasing anemia, increasing numbers of basophils, more marrow blasts and promyelocytes, new chromosomal abnormalities, chloromas, increasing myelofibrosis or spleen size, new systemic symptoms (fevers, sweats, bone pain, weight loss), lymphadenopathy, and hypercalcemia have all been reported as heralding an AP. Patients may then progress to BC, which is acute leukemia-type picture. Most cases of BC are myeloid in origin, but 20% may be lymphoid, and a few will be megakaryocytic.

10. CLL is most often staged by the Rai classification:
    Stage 0: lymphocytosis $> 15,000$/mm^3
    Stage I: lymphocytosis and lymphadenopathy
    Stage II: lymphocytosis with an enlarged spleen or liver
    Stage III: lymphocytosis with anemia (autoimmune or decreased production)
    Stage IV: lymphocytosis with thrombocytopenia, anemia and lymphadenopathy

11. The goal of treatment in the chronic phase of CML is to "control" the WBC and try to normalize as much as possible the levels of hemoglobin, red cells, and platelets. Hydroxyurea is now the preferred agent, although busulfan may also be used. New studies show that alpha-

interferon may be effective in this phase, and in some cases, the Ph1 positive clone "disappears" from the marrow with this treatment.

12. Accelerated phase and acute phase are more difficult to treat (and treatment is less effective). Acute leukemia regimens are used for BC, and those with lymphoblastic type blasts have a "better" prognosis.

13. The use of allogenic bone marrow transplantation in chronic phase is exciting. Identical twin transplants albeit rare are highly effective.

14. CLL is treated with oral alkylating agents like chlorambucil or cyclophosphamide. These are reserved for patients with Rai stage III or IV. A new agent called fludarabine has shown promising results.

15. For HCL, two agents, interferon and deoxycoformycin, have been highly effective.

LIVER (HEPATOCELLULAR) CANCER

1. Most often presents with right upper quadrant or epigastric pain, an increase or appearance of ascites or an unexplained deterioration in the course of a patient with cirrhosis.

2. Always think about hemochromatosis as predisposing event. Family members can be screened.

3. The alpha-fetoprotein is elevated in 80% of cases.

4. The tumor may present with polycythemia (secondary to erythroprotein), hypercalcemia (due to PTH-like substance), hypoglycemia, abnormal coagulation tests (including dysfibrinogenemia), or an elevated B_{12} level or male feminization.

5. The only curative treatment is surgery, but the resectability rate is less than 30%.

6. Radiation may help to control capsular pain.

7. Chemotherapy has limited usefulness.

8. Direct hepatic artery infusion may produce more responses and possibly, longer survival.

9. New approaches include radioactive isotopes which "home" to the surface of the hepatocellular carcinoma (like a Trojan horse) and chemoembolization using concomitant chemotherapeutic drug and a particle which causes vascular flow arrest. Other new approaches can be assessed through the literature searches mentioned in chapter 20.

LUNG CANCER

1. Lung cancer is the leading cause of cancer death in the United States in both men and women and is rapidly becoming the number one cancer in the world.

2. Symptoms may be due to tumor growth at the primary site (e.g., cough, hemoptysis, dyspnea, obstructive pneumonitis, or chest wall pain); symptoms due to regional spread (e.g., hoarseness due to recurrent laryngeal nerve involvement, SVC syndrome, or pericardial encroachment); symptoms due to metastatic spread to any one of a number of organs, the most common being the brain, bones, liver, adrenal glands, and lymph nodes; and finally, due to paraneoplastic effects caused by substances, most commonly hormones secreted by the tumor.

    Typically, there is about a three month delay before a patient seeks medical advice after developing symptoms, and about the same time delay before the physician finally makes the diagnosis.

3. Every effort must be made to get a diagnosis. Cytology is adequate, but histology is preferable. Choice of appropriate test to obtain tissue depends on the location of the tumor mass, i.e., in the center or the periphery of the chest. Prebiopsy tests should include careful history and physical exam, screening laboratory tests such as CBC, alkaline phosphatase, SGOT, calcium, sodium, potassium, and routine chest x-ray. Specialized x-ray procedures such as CAT scans or MRI's may add additional information about tumor location, relationship to adjacent structures, metastases to mediastinum, liver, adrenals, or retroperitoneal structures. Tissue procurement may include: a) sputum cytology on three occasions (best done in the morning when secretions have pooled overnight. HINTS: seek help from the respiratory therapists to obtain a good specimen and always get a specimen after bronchoscopy—this "stirs up" the epithelium and may be associated with a better specimen); b) bronchoscopy with biopsies, cytology, and

bronchial washings; c) needle aspiration cytology (usually performed percutaneously for peripheral lesions; d) mediastinoscopy or mediastinotomy on the left side because of the arch of the aorta. Thoracotomy is not generally used as the first diagnostic procedure to obtain a tissue diagnosis, but may be used in small, peripheral lesions in which staging procedures fail to reveal metastases.

4. Several cell types are seen in lung cancer, each with some differences in behavior and patterns of disease. These details are important as they often carry significance in decision making during diagnosis, staging, and treatment selection. Important points to remember are: a) Small cell carcinoma (20–25%) has frequent spread of gross or microscopic disease, is rarely treated with surgery, and is often associated with paraneoplastic hormonal syndromes (e.g. SIADH, ectopic ACTH production) b) Well-differentiated squamous cell carcinoma tends to be more "slowly" growing and less often will spread beyond regional lymph nodes, c) All other "non-small cell" cancers (i.e. adenocarcinoma, large cell carcinoma, and poorly differentiated squamous cell carcinoma) behave in a similar manner with a greater tendency to produce metastases than those tumors listed in b.

5. Prior to surgery, it is necessary to adequately stage the patient. One goal of staging is to determine whether the patient (in categories 4b and c above) is a candidate for "curative" therapy. i.e. surgery and in some cases, radiation. Treatment selection will also depend on other physiologic parameters such as respiratory and cardiovascular function (can the patient withstand an aggressive "curative" approach?).

Staging procedures include all of the tests listed in 3 above i.e., H&P, labs, CXR, CT scan of the chest, liver, adrenals, and upper abdomen. Other tests include a bone scan, which is more likely to be helpful if there are bone symptoms or an elevated alkaline phosphatase, and a CT scan of the brain. Many argue against the utility of these latter two tests. They should always be done in staging patients with small cell carcinoma, and you should discuss the philosophy of doing these tests in your institution with the diagnostic radiologists and thoracic surgeons. In small cell patients, a bone marrow should also be done.

One of the most important staging tests is the mediastinoscopy. If mediastinal nodes are involved, for all practical purposes, the patient is inoperable (exception below).

6. With the exception of small cell carcinoma, the primary treatment is surgery if at all possible. The following lists reasons for inoperability:

> Paralyzed vocal cord or diaphragm
> Esophageal involvement
> Atelectasis or obstructive pneumonia of an entire lung
> Pleural effusion
> Horner's syndrome
> SVC syndrome
> Pericardial effusion or cardiac involvement
> Severe lung disease or pulmonary hypertension
> Tumor in trachea or less than 2cm. from carina
> Medical condition precluding pulmonary surgery
> Spread outside the chest or to the mediastinum

In some cases of ipsilateral nodes low in the mediatinum, surgery may be feasible with "good" results. Also, tumors that invade the chest wall or ribs may be resected, especially when surgery is combined with radiation.

For localized tumors in which resection is not feasible, or if the patient refuses, radiation is a viable option. The median survival for patients receiving "curative" radiation is over a year, but some patients achieve a long term "complete" remission. Some current programs are combining radiation with chemotherapy and even surgery with some promising results.

7. Small cell carcinoma is approached entirely differently. With the exception of a few tumors located in the lung periphery, most of these patients have bulky disease at the primary site. About half of patients at presentation have demonstrable disease found outside the chest on the staging procedures. The philosophy is that ALL patients will have microscopic disease outside the chest and some form of systemic therapy is necessary. Chemotherapy has become the primary treatment modality with a number of combinations of drugs showing a beneficial effect. Response rates of 50–90% are seen In patients with disease encompassible by a radiation port (so called limited stage disease), and radiation added to the chemotherapy improves both survival and control of the disease within the chest. The CNS is also treated "prophylactically" with radiation to prevent growth in this frequent metastatic site which may not "see" appropriate concentrations of chemotherapy because of the blood-brain barrier.

8. Overall survival has remained between 5–10% despite improvements in the therapy for small cell and improved post-operative support for those patients with other types. For operable cases, the outlook is slightly better with 30–50% of early stage cases surviving 5 years.

9. Lung cancer produces a wide range of hormonal and neurologic syndromes. In squamous cell carcinoma, hypercalcemia predominates. A parathyroid-like hormone (which is not PTH) has been implicated. Cases are also seen of peripheral neuropathy, cerebellar degeneration, dermatomyositis and pulmonary hypertrophic osteoarthropathy. In small cell, hormonal syndromes predominate (e.g. SIADH, or ectopic ACTH). Other syndromes include the Eaton-Lambert syndrome, a neurologic disorder causing defective release of acetylcholine at the neuromuscular junction. Many neuroendocrine markers have been measured in the serum of patients with small cell, but none have yet had a practical application in the management of this disease.

10. Lung cancer is too common and too lethal. The tragedy is that it is also one of the most preventable. Work to get your patients to stop or never start smoking!

LYMPHOMAS: HODGKIN'S DISEASE

1. Hodgkin's disease represents a real "success" story in the management of cancer. The introduction of MOPP chemotherapy by DeVita not only produced cures in what used to be uniformly fatal late stage Hodgkin's, but also changed the slope of the cancer death rate curves for young people and spawned the optimism for combination chemotherapy that marked the past two decades.

2. Hodgkin's usually presents with swollen lymph nodes, most commonly in the neck. Symptoms include fevers, drenching night sweats, and weight loss of >10% (these three symptoms are the so-called "B" symptoms). There also may be the unusual symptom of pain in lymph node areas with consumption of alcohol.

   Recently, cases of Hodgkin's are being seen in patients with AIDS, and these cases present with infiltrates in the lungs or skin which is a most unusual presentation for Hodgkin's in the non-immunocompromised host.

3. The diagnosis is made from examination of the lymph node (or other tissue) and the finding of the malignant cell—the Reed-Sternberg cell—in the appropriate milieu. The pathologist often sees replacement of a node with normal, reactive eosinophils, lymphocytes, and plasma cells. This type of background makes the pathologist look carefully for the R-S cells. There are four histologic subtypes of Hodgkin's: lymphocyte predominant, nodular sclerosing, mixed cellularity, and lymphocyte depleted. These are listed in descending order of prognosis.

4. Hodgkin's has four stages, each divided into "A" and "B" representing those without or with the symptoms mentioned above.

   Stage 1 represents one lymph node group involved on one side of the diaphragm. Stage 2 represents two or more groups involved, but on the same side of the diaphragm. Stage 3 represents involvement on both sides of the diaphragm. Stage 4 represents disease outside the nodes (the spleen is considered a "node" and the subscript "s" denotes splenic involvement). The subscript "E" connotes direct extension from a node into contiguous tissue.

   A stage is assigned to be able to tell the patient about prognosis, to be able to decide how to treat and to be able to compare studies.

5. Staging procedures include:
   a) A careful H&P
   b) Labs—CBC, liver tests
   c) CXR, and CT to define the mediastinum if suspicious
   d) Bilateral bone marrow biopsy
   e) Abdominal imaging, i.e. CT, ultrasound and/or lymphangiogram
   f) Exploratory laparotomy
      (if it will change therapy)

6. Conventional treatment is radiation for stages 1–3A (total nodal radiation) and combination chemotherapy for stages 3B and 4A or B.

   Combinations of chemotherapy and radiation are being tested in lower stage patients who might have poor prognostic signs.

7. Complications of radiation include second malignancies in the fields treated and the sequellae of radiation fibrosis in the organs treated (e.g. hypothyroidism or pulmonary fibrosis). Combined modality therapy has been associated with the development of acute leukemia in about 4% of patients. There also is an increased incidence of non-Hodgkin's lymphoma. MOPP chemotherapy is associated with sterility.

LYMPHOMAS: NON-HODGKIN'S

1. These constitute some of the most difficult to understand diseases in oncology, but they are also one of the most exciting and rewarding groups of diseases to treat. NHL account for about 75% of the lymphomas.

2. The major differences between Hodgkin's and NHL are:
   NHL patients are much more likely to have extranodal primaries (e.g. in the stomach or thyroid)
   NHL patients are much more likely to have lymph nodes in the periphery of the body involved, in contrast to Hodgkin's which almost always involves nodes in the center of the body (e.g. paraaortics vs mesenterics in NHL)
   NHL patients are much more likely to have "skip" areas, whereas Hodgkin's usually involves contiguous nodal groups. These latter two points make nodal radiation a rational treatment for Hodgkin's, but much less useful for NHL.

3. The classification systems are many and varied. The most commonly used one is the International Working Formulation.
   A. Low grade lymphomas
      1) Small lymphocytic (SL)
      2) Follicular, small cleaved cell (FSC)
      3) Follicular, mixed small cleaved and large cell (FM)
   B. Intermediate-grade lymphomas
      4) Follicular, large cell (FL)
      5) Diffuse, small cleaved cell (DSC)
      6) Diffuse, mixed, small and large cell (DM)
      7) Diffuse, large cell, cleaved/noncleaved (DL)
   C. High-grade lymphomas
      8) Diffuse, large cell, immunoblastic (IBL)
      9) Lymphoblastic convoluted/nonconvoluted (LBL)
      10) Small, noncleaved cell, Burkitt's (SNC)
      11) Miscellaneous
          Composite
          Mycosis fungoides (Sezary)
          Histiocytic
          Extramedullary plasmacytoma
          Other

Many physicians still use the Rapoport system. Rapoport substitutes nodular for follicular. It also calls the large cell types "histiocytic" instead of recognizing that these large cells are lymphocytes.

An oncology fellow training at our institution classified the A, B, and C categories above as "the good, the bad, and the ugly."

4. Symptoms, signs and staging are similar to that discussed in the Hodgkin's section with the exception that alcohol associated pain is more common in Hodgkin's. NHL patients are much more likely to have higher stage disease at presentation, and very infrequently, would require a laparotomy for staging.

5. The low grade group have long natural histories, may sometimes spontaneously regress, are often first treated by "watchful waiting" and when they require treatment, gentle, oral therapy is often used. One of the paradoxes of the lymphomas is that these low grade ones can almost never be cured, while their more aggressive cousins can often be cured by very aggressive therapy. The intermediate and high grade groups are treated with high doses of multi-agent chemotherapy, and greater than 50% are cured.

6. If the bowel is the primary site, and a resection is possible, it is the preferred therapy, since perforation due to rapid lysis of the sensitive cells may occur. Chemotherapy after surgery is very effective at preventing relapses.

7. HTLV-1 is currently the only definitive human cancer causing retrovirus. It causes a rare T cell lymphoma, often associated with skin infiltration and hypercalcemia.

MALIGNANT MELANOMA (Cutaneous)

1. Melanoma is second only to lung cancer in females as the most rapidly rising cancer in the U.S. The etiology is unquestionably related to u.v. light exposure, and with increased leisure time, different clothing habits, and possibly, depletion of the protective ozone layer, the incidence of melanoma is rising.

2. The dysplastic nevus syndrome is a relatively recently described preneoplastic condition. Reference to an excellent atlas of these lesions is given in Chapter 5.

3. Chapter 5 also describes the early signs of malignancy in a pigmented lesion which include: a variegated color, a notch in the border, asymmetry, and a change in a lesion.

4. Excisional biopsy of a suspicious lesion is preferred. Refer suspicious lesions to a dermatologist. Many institutions have established a pigmented lesions clinic.

5. Melanomas are divided into three stages:
   Stage I = a localized lesion.
   Stage II = regional nodes.
   Stage III = distant metastases.
   Stage I is subclassified by depth of invasion. There are two classifications: Clark's and Breslow's.
   Clark's levels are:
   Level I = entirely within the epidermis.
   Level II = into papillary dermis.
   Level III = at border of papillary and reticular dermis.
   Level IV = into reticular dermis.
   Level V = into subcutaneous fat.
   Breslow simply measured the depth of invasion in millimeters. The deeper the invasion (or the higher the Clark's level), the worse the prognosis (i.e. the more chance of nodal or distant disease).
   Breslow's level less than 0.76 mm have an excellent prognosis after excision.

6. Primary treatment involves a wide excision of the lesion (2–5 cm margins with skin graft if necessary to achieve closure), but if the melanoma is ≤1 mm in depth, 1 cm. margins are acceptable.
   The value of a regional lymph node dissection is currently under investigation, as previous randomized, controlled trials have shown no definite benefit for prophylactic dissections; yet certain subsets (intermediate thickness) may fare better with dissection.

7. Melanoma is generally considered radiation-resistant but altered time-dose fractionation with high, twice weekly dosing may provide palliation.
   DTIC (which has a 15–20% response rate) is the traditional mainstay of chemotherapy treatment for metastases (responses are more likely to occur in soft tissue or nodal disease, rather than in visceral metastases).

Combinations such as DTIC, cisplatinum, BCNL
have shown higher anti-tumor activity.

- Immunologic interventions with some successes inclu
  tralesional injections lead to regressions in 60%, and
  regressions of distant disease too), alpha interferon, and
  cells, both of which have about a 20% response rate.
- Surgical excision of single metastases is acceptable, especially if
  there is a long disease free interval, or if symptomatic (e.g.
  pain).

8. Melanoma is the most common tumor to spontaneously regress. It is
the most common solid tumor to metastasize to the spleen. It also
metastasizes to the heart, and GI tract more frequently than other
tumors.

Those with soft tissue or nodal metastases do better. Pulmonary
metastases are intermediate in prognosis and other visceral metastases
more grim in their prognostic significance.

MULTIPLE MYELOMA

1. Multiple Myeloma (MM) is a malignant clonal disorder of plasma cells.
In 99% of cases, the cells secrete complete or parts of (light chains)
immunoglobulins producing a serum or urine "M" protein. MM should
be contrasted with Waldenstrom's macroglobulinemia (WM), an IgM
secreting tumor of plasmacytoid lymphocytes. The following table contrasts the differences between these two diseases, and also includes
monoclonal gammopathy of undetermined significance (MGUS). 1% of
people at age 50 have a small "M spike" found on protein electropho-
resis, 3% at 70 and 12% at 90. For most of these people, this lab
phenomenon has no significance to their health.

	MM	*WM*	*MGUS*
Cell	Plasma	Plasmacytoid lymph	May be increased in "normal" plasma cells
Protein	IgG—50%	IgM	<2.5 gm

	MM	*WM*	*MGUS*
	IgA—25% IgD, E-rare Bence-Jones—25% proteins (light chains) Nonsecretors—1% (have decrease in normal Ig's)	BJP—25%	IgG, no decrease in normal immunoglobins
Bone	Lytic: 2/3, osteoporosis	Rare (5%)	0
Calcium	High in 10%	Usually normal	Normal
Renal	Abnl in 50%	Abnl in 33%	Normal
Hyperviscosity	30–50%	Uncommon (IgA.IgG)	0

2. Diagnostic criteria for MM include:
Major criteria
a) Tissue plasmacytoma
b) >30% plasma cells in marrow
c) >3.5gm/dl IgG or >2gm/dl IgA monoclonal M components; >1gm/ 24 hr excretion of lambda or kappa light chains in the urine
Minor criteria
a) 10–30% plasma cells in the bone marrow
b) Monoclonal M component or urinary light chain excretion at lower levels than above
c) Skeletal lytic lesions
d) Serum (normal polyclonal) IgM<50mg/dl, IgA<100mg/dl, IgG<600 mg/dl

One major and one minor criterion, or three minor criteria, one of which must be increased plasma cells in the marrow and a monoclonal spike, establish a diagnosis of myeloma.

Beta-2 macroglobulin levels have recently been shown to be a prognostic factor and useful as a marker to follow the disease.

3. Prognostic factors include: level and type of "M" protein, presence of renal failure or hypercalcemia, and degree of bony lesions. In general, nonsecretory tumors are the worst, and patients whose IgG levels>7gm, IgA>5 and BJP>12 have worse prognoses. IgD myeloma is often associated with amyloid deposition.

4. Complications of MM include:

   a) Renal failure which may be caused by light chain destruction of the proximal tubules causing a Fanconi-like syndrome (this is called myeloma kidney), hypercalcemia, hyperuricemia, infection, amyloid, or an obstructing plasmacytoma. Careful hydration should be given if patients are to receive contrast agents which may precipitate acute tubular necrosis.

   b) Infection which is in part due to low levels of the normal immunoglobulins and lowered white counts due to disease infiltration of the marrow as well as the effects of therapy.

   c) Anemia and thrombocytopenia due to disease and therapy. The platelets may also have qualitative defects due to rthe coating immunoglobulins. Rouleux formation is frequently seen on the peripheral smear.

   d) Bone destruction, both lytic lesions and osteoporosis. Bone compression and severe pain and deformity are common.

   e) Hypercalcemia due to the production of osteoclast activating factor.

5. The usual first treatment is melphalan plus prednisone. Refractory cases have recently been given the combination of vincristine, adriamycin plus dexamethasone with some success. High dose therapies with autologous bone marrow "rescues" are being attempted.

OSTEOSARCOMA

1. Osteosarcoma is most commonly a neoplasm of childhood and adolescence characterized by malignant spindle cell appearance associated with osteoid production. (Included in this spindle cell group are also malignant fibrous histiocytoma and fibrosarcoma.) Knee joint and lesions of the proximal humerus account for 25–50% of cases. There is biologic evidence that the malignant cell has lost both alleles of the "RB" (retinoblastoma) gene on chromosome 13 (thus loss of a protective effect on cell growth by a so-called antioncogene).

2. Pain is most common presenting complaint. Tenderness and a soft tissue mass fixed to bone are often found on a physical examination.

3. Radiographic signs include periosteal elevation, cortical destruction, and extraosseous extension. The alkaline phosphatase level is elevated in 50% of cases. There is a poorer prognosis if > 2 aneuploid cell lines in tumor, DNA index > 2.0, or S phase fraction > 12%.

4. The lung is the most common site for metastasis. Work up includes CXR, MRI or CT of the bone, CT scan of chest, and routine chemistries.

5. Historically amputation one joint above tumor containing bone was the treatment of choice, but now alternatives for limb-sparing surgery are available. Separate lung nodules (some say up to 15) may be considered resectable with median sternotomy. Neoadjuvant chemotherapy is now often given.

6. Active chemotherapeutic agents include cisplatinum, doxorubicin, methotrexate (high dose) and with preoperative treatment > 50% are in complete remission at the time of operation. Tumors found to be of higher grade are generally given preop and/or postop chemotherapy. Ifosfamide is a promising new agent with up to 60% responding, even if refractory to prior chemotherapy.

OVARIAN CANCER

1. Ovarian cancer is the major cause of death in gynecological cancers with approximately 19,000 new cases annually in the U.S. (1 woman in 70 will develop in her lifetime) The peak incidence occurs between age 40 and 70.

2. Generally, it presents with vague abdominal or pelvic complaints (e.g. "indigestion", bloating, nausea, "aching"); increase in girth, typically indicates ascites. Palpable ovary in a post-menopausal woman is cause for concern.

3. An ultrasound or CT scan will usually demonstrate ovarian mass with or without ascites CA-125 is an antigen present in nonmucinous ovarian carcinomas, and occasionally in other non-gynecologic carcinomas, and in 1% of healthy individuals. If the levels are > 35 units/ml , this is a strong indicator of potential ovarian neoplasm. An exploratory laparotomy is warranted in most cases to confirm the diagnosis and

assess extent of disease. The entire abdominal cavity must be explored since metastases often "hide" in the upper abdomen.

4. The work up should include CXR, routine lab; barium enema, and sigmoid oscopy. An IVP is also often done.

5. Staging (in brief)

    I. Growth limited to ovaries

    II. Growth in one or both ovaries with pelvic extension

    III. Peritoneal implants outside the pelvis and/or positive retroperitoneal or inguinal nodes

    IV. Distant metastasis

The grade of the tumor also affects prognosis.

6. The primary treatment is total abdominal hysterectomy and bilateral salpingo-oophorectomy, omentectomy, multiple biopsies of peritoneal surface, and lymph nodes. If clinical Stage I in young woman, a unilateral salpingo-oophorectomy is permissible. Debulking all sites of tumor (if technically feasible) to <1.5 cm (as largest remaining mass) appears to confer a better prognosis.

7. If Stage I with favorable tumor grade or if borderline malignancy, there is no benefit to adding chemotherapy or radiation therapy. If Stage I, with unfavorable grade, follow-up chemotherapy (e.g. 6 cycles of "CAP")or radiation therapy is utilized.

8. Since the majority of patients are Stage III at diagnosis, chemotherapy is a mainstay of treatment (cisplatinum 100–150 mg/m^2 IV or carboplatin 300–400 mg/m^2 IV repeated at 3–4 week intervals for 4–6 cycles) with or without cyclophosphamide and Adriamycin. Other active agents include ifosfamide, Taxol, hexamethylmelamine.

9. Intraperitoneal chemotherapy or immunotherapy (interferon, interleukin-2, monoclonal antibodies) is being investigated.

10. Second look laparotomies are often done especially in research programs, where assessment of response is crucial. A CA-125 level > 35 u/ml accurately predicts relapse.

PANCREATIC CANCER

1. This is the fourth most common cause of cancer death and the incidence is rising in the U.S., especially in Alaska. There is a 2% 5-year survival.

2. 80% involve the head of pancreas and 20% involve the body or tail. Most are ductal adenocarcinomas (75%) with <5% adenosquamos or acinar cells. Cystadenocarcinomas account for about 1%, and have a better prognosis.

3. Pancreatic cancer tends to grow silently and invade extensively into local tissues before diagnosis can be made. There are no effective screening tests.

4. 95% of patients present with one or more of these symptoms, weight loss, jaundice, pain. Other findings can include a palpable mass, a palpable gallbladder (20%) or a paraneoplastic syndrome like "migratory thrombrophlebitis."

5. Diagnostic tests:
   a. Ultrasound or CT, usually will show mass and/or dilated ducts.
   b. ERCP with cytology if available or transhepatic cholangiography.
   c. Attempts should be made to make a tissue diagnosis by aspiration cytology if available.

6. The treatment is dismal.
   a. Only about 15% of patients are candidates for attempts at curative surgery.
   b. The operative mortality of a Whipple type operation is 10–30% and the 5 year survival only 15%.
   c. National groups have added radiation and chemotherapy to those patients with resections and there seems to be a slight survival increase (? survival of the fittest).
   d. Palliative surgery to relieve jaundice should be contemplated.
   e. Radiation may help palliate pain, but often not. Appropriate use of analgesics is essential.
   f. Current chemotherapy has not proven to be of much benefit.

7. Future possibilities include the use of intraoperative radiation combined with hyperthermia. Consult the databases in Chapter 20 for other new developments.

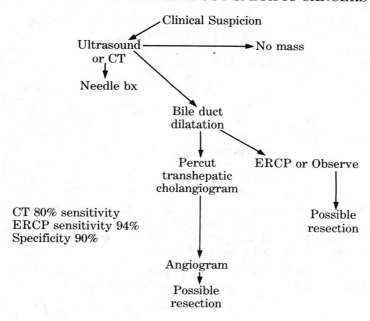

CT 80% sensitivity
ERCP sensitivity 94%
Specificity 90%

8. Islet Cell Tumors

Native Hormone Secretion

Hormone	*Tumor*	*Therapy*
Insulin	Insulinoma	Diazoxide
Glucagon	Glucagonoma	
Somatostatin	Somatostatinoma	

Ectopic Hormone Secretion

Hormone	*Syndrome*	*Therapy*
Gastrin	Zollinger-Ellison	Cimetidine
Vasoactive intestinal polypeptide	Watery diarrhea, hypokalemia, achlorhydria	
Prostaglandin E	WDHA	Indomethacin
ACTH/CRH	Cushing's	

Hormone	Syndrome	Therapy
MSH	Hyperpigmentation	
Serotonin	Carcinoid	
Chorionic gonadotrophin	Precocious puberty, gynecomastia	
ADH	SIADH	Water restriction, dimechlocycline, lithium

PROSTATE CANCER

1. The mortality rate for prostate cancer has been constant for the last thirty years. Almost half of the patients present with stage D disease.

2. Attempts at early detection are in progress (discussed in Chapter 5). Transrectal ultrasound and the new serum marker prostate specific antigen may be useful in detecting non-palpable tumors. These tests are too non-specific and insensitive though.

3. Prostate cancer is divided into four stages: A, B, C, and D. The following table lists the definitions, and staging tests.

Positive Stage	Acid P'tase	Bone Scan	LN's at Dissection
A. Tumor is not palpable—detected at TURP			
A_1 involves <5% of specimen (low grade)	NL	NL	<5%
A_2 involves >5% (high grade)	NL	NL	25%
B. Nodule palpable			
B_1 no more than half of 1 lobe	NL	NL	10–15%
B_2 more than half of 1 lobe	NL	NL	30%
B_3 more than 1 lobe (not all staging systems use B_3)			
C extends outside capsule	may be elevated	NL	45%
D outside gland			
D_1 pelvic lymph	may be elevated	NL	
D_2 bone metastasis	often elevated	+	

The last column shows how the disease is understaged. When lymph node dissections are done, many more patients actually have D_1 disease.

4. One important prognostic factor is the grade. Gleason has devised a system whereby the worst and second worst areas are graded on a scale of 1 to 5. Both scores are added to give a total—the higher the number, the more aggressive the behavior of the cancer.

5. Treatment:
   A_1 Observation   (2% progress)
   A_2, $B_{1,2}$ Consideration of radical prostatectomy versus radiation
   C   Radiation

   When making a decision, one must take into careful consideration the age and performance status of the patient. If the expected lifespan is less than 5 years, aggressive local treatment may not be indicated. Surgery is favored in stage B disease.

Complications of Radical Prostatectomy and Radiation

Complication	Radical Prostatectomy	RT
Urinary incontinence	Occasionally	Rare
Bladder neck contracture	Occasionally	Occasionally
Impotence	Almost invariable*	Frequent
Cystitis	Rare	Occasionally
Urethral stricture	Rare	Occasionally
Dermatitis	Never	Rare
Proctitis	Never	Occasionally
Lymphocoeles	Occasionally	Never
Comorbid comps.	Occasionally	Rare

*There is now a nerve-sparing operation developed by Walsh at Johns Hopkins in which 80% of patients maintain potency.

7. The PSA post-op may be more useful in following disease status than it is in the screening situation.

8. Stage D disease responds to hormonal treatment with palliation of symptoms in most patients.

   First line therapy should be either orchiectomy or LHRH—agonists. The latter have few side effects (except hot flashes and decreased libido), but they are costly ($300.00–$400.00/month). Monthly depot injections have been developed.

Second line therapy could include: orchiectomy (if not done first), or flutamide 250mg tid (an antiandrogen—cost $210.00/month). Other hormonal treatments that have been used include Megace 40 mg tid, ketoconazole (400 mg tid), aminoglutethamide 250 mg. tid. both of which block adrenal steroidogenesis. Second line treatments rarely are effective.

9. There is a great deal of excitement about combined hormonal blockage (complete androgen ablation) using orchiectomy or LHRH—A plus flutamide. Recent data from controlled trials show this therapy to be marginally better than single agents. Use in earlier stage disease (B & C) seems promising.

10. It is difficult to assess the use of chemotherapeutic agents in prostate cancer because of the difficulty in measuring objective criteria for response. The most effective agents appear to be cytoxan and cisplatin.

11. There is a great deal of excitement about suramin which inhibits certain growth factors.

12. Once metastatic, the key to therapy is effective palliation with attention to the quality of life. Stepwise, sequential hormonal manipulation and judicious use of radiation are the cornerstones of therapy.

SOFT TISSUE SARCOMAS

1. There are many different types of malignant tumors arising in connective tissue that are grouped because of similarities in behavior and appearance.

   There are approximately 5000 new cases annually in U.S.and certain genetic syndromes may predispose (e.g. neurofibromatosis, tuberous sclerosis, and the basal cell nevus syndrome).

2. They usually present as a mass with or without pain.

3. The diagnosis is made by generous incisional (or if small, excisional) biopsy. Accurate assessment of grade is very important. The location of biopsy site is crucial in order not to interfere with later therapeutic excision.

   Electron microscopy may be helpful for delineating those tumors likely to behave more aggressively.

4. Appropriate diagnostic studies include xerograms of soft tissue components, and CT scan, or MRI to delineate tissue planes. An arteriogram is often valuable in planning surgery.

   A CT of chest (or tomograms) is done to evaluate for distant metastases. A bone scan is done to evaluate for for possible involvement regionally by the primary mass.

5. Surgical excision with negative margins is the cornerstone of treatment, and amputation may be necessary.

   Radiation therapy alone is not very effective due to the high dose requirement for these relatively insensitive tumors, but when combined with surgery, can achieve local control in 80–90%.

   Adjuvant chemotherapy—active agents: doxorubicin, DTIC, cyclophosphamide, methotrexate-may be beneficial for sarcomas arising in an extremity.

6. Lung metastases may be resectable, if no other metastases are found outside of chest and the primary site is controlled.

   Doxorubicin 70 mg/m^2 IV and DTIC 1 gram/m^2 IV divided over 2 days are considered the standard agents. Ifosfamide is also an effective agent.

7. The therapy of sarcomas is highly sophisticated and undergoing rapid change. Consult the electronic data bases for any patient for the most up-to-date therapy (see Chapter 20).

STOMACH CANCER

1. There has been a marked decrease in the incidence of stomach cancer is over the past half-century. It is now the eighth most common cancer in the U.S. and accounts for 20,000 new cases per year. Because of its continued high rates in other parts of the world, particularly the Orient, and because second generation migrants have rates similar to the host country, environmental causes are likely etiologic agents, particularly diet.

2. It is speculated that decreased consumption of smoked and pickled foods may lead to decreased exposure to nitrosamines and polycyclic hydrocarbons. Vitamin C may also protect. Gastroscopy has been practiced in areas of high risk, but its value is not clear.

3. No specific set of symptoms has been seen and symptoms and signs can vary from vague abdominal distress, to anemia, to signs of meta-

static disease with palpable masses and ascites. Depending on location, it may present with signs of gastric outlet obstruction. Significant anorexia with distaste for meat is frequently seen. Hematemesis is unusual as a presenting sign.

4. Diagnostic workup should include an upper gastrointestinal series followed by a gastroscopy if there is a suspicious ulcer, a polypoid mass seen, or a lesion with characteristics of linitus plastica.

5. Four histologic patterns are seen: ulcerative, polypoid, scirrhous or linitis plastica, and superficial. These are related to the degree of differentiation of the tumor, with linitis plastica having the worst prognosis.

6. Staging tests include routine laboratory tests, chest x-ray and abdominal CT scan. In addition, careful examination of the pelvis to rule out involvement of the ovaries (Krukenberg tumors) or the area above the rectum (Blumer's shelf) should be performed.

7. Surgical resection of the stomach with adequate surgical margins must be obtained. This may involve a subtotal or total gastrectomy. Removal of the first echelon of nodes has been advocated, though recent studies suggest that the second echelon of nodes should also be removed. Adjuvant radiation therapy with or without chemotherapy probably has a role to play in trying to prevent loco-regional relapse. Adjuvant chemotherapy has not been effective.

8. Only a small fraction of patients with stomach cancer are cured using locally aggressive therapy and most will develop metastatic disease. Treatment of metastatic disease with chemotherapy has had a limited impact upon survival, but may in the individual patient provide some benefit. The standard therapy is 5-flurouracil, Adriamycin, mitomycin C (FAM), with response rates averaging about 30–40%. Newer protocols include VP-16 and platinum.

9. Paraneoplastic syndromes include microangiopathic hemolytic anemia (which can also occur as a complication of mitomycin C therapy), thrombophlebitis in multiple sites, and marantic endocarditis.

TESTICULAR CANCER

1. Testicular cancer is the most common cancer in males during the third decade of life (5700 new cases/year). Combined treatment with sur-

gery and chemotherapy have improved the cure rate to well over 90%. Radiation therapy combined with surgery is curative in almost 100% of seminomas.

2. Testicular self-exam has been advocated in young males, but its efficacy has not been proven.

3. A "mass" in the testicle (occasionally associated with pain) is the primary symptom. There is usually a long delay before seeking medical care. All young males should have an M.D. exam at the time of their physical exams.

4. Physical examination by a urologist, followed by an ultrasound examination of the affected testis will detect suspicious masses. If there is a solid suspicious mass, it should be removed. Transscrotal biopsy should not be performed as it raises the risk of scrotal contamination (the lymphatic drainage is different from the scrotum and would complicate treatment planning if radiation therapy were to be used. A radial inguinal orchiectomy is the procedure of choice.

5. Serum markers, human chorionic gonadotrophin and alpha-feto-protein should be obtained prior to and after surgery. Pretherapy, or immediately after the inguinal orchiectomy performed for diagnosis and treatment of the localized tumor, a CT scan of the abdomen and pelvis to determine the size of the retroperitoneal lymph nodes and a chest x-ray to rule out metastases to the lungs should be performed. Treatment planning will depend on the stage of the disease. If the retroperitoneal nodes are negative or minimally involved a nerve sparing retroperitoneal lymph node dissection should be performed.

6. Most tumors (95%) are of germ cell origin. Those of stromal origin (e.g. Leydig cell tumors and Sertoli cell tumors) will not be discussed.

   The germ cell tumors are divided into seminomas, and non-seminomas which include choriocarcinomas, embryonal cell carcinomas, endodermal sinus tumors, and teratomas. 40% are mixtures of several cell types.

   The markers are related to the histology as follows:

   Choriocarcinoma—produces B-HCG: (some seminomas with syncytial trophoblastic giant cells can produce HCG, but these should be treated as seminomas)

   Embryonal cell tumors produce AFP.

   Endodermal sinus tumors produce both markers.

   Teratomas may produce AFP.

Even if one doesn't see the element listed above histologically, it is there (e.g. in a metastasis) and should be treated as such The half-life of HCG is 24 hours, and AFP, 6 days. If the markers don't return to normal after therapy or begin to rise, tumor is still present and should be treated as such.

7. A radical inguinal orchiectomy must be performed to control the primary tumor. If the patient has a non-seminomatous germ cell cancer, a retroperitoneal lymph node dissection should be performed to further stage the patient and define those who should receive immediate chemotherapy. (This has been controversial in the past, with some investigators following the patient with serial markers and CT scans of the retroperitoneum. Controlled trials now show that patients will die of their disease using this more conservative approach.)

8. Chemotherapy given to those patients with positive nodes should bring the cure rate to nearly 100%. Current guidelines indicate that two cycles of etoposide (VP-16), bleomycin, and cisplatin should be given.

9. In patients with pure seminomas confined to the testes, prophylactic radiation to the retroperitoneum should be given. In patients with metastatic disease several chemotherapy regiments have high complete response and cure rates. Vinblastine or VP-16, bleomycin, and cisplatin are the primary treatment regimens, but salvage regimens may include these drugs plus ifosphamide and/or adriamycin. In some cases after successful treatment with chemotherapy, further surgical removal of remaining tumor nodules may be beneficial. Sometimes these surgical specimens show residual malignant tumor, but also, they may show benign tumors or fibrosis.

10. Using current treatment approaches potency and fertility should be preserved. Prior to nerve sparing node dissections, a high rate of retrograde ejaculation resulted in infertility. The current drug programs may cause temporary sterility, and if the physician or patient have any worries about this, sperm banking prior to node dissection and chemotherapy should be considered. (However, patients with testicular cancer have been shown to have abnormal sperm counts and motility even prior to therapy.)

11. Germ cells reach the embryonic testes from their origin in yolk sac by migrating up the midline to the urogenital ridge. Sometimes they

"miss" and residual nests of germ cells may be found in the midline stuctures like the pineal gland or the mediastinum. Young men with tumors of these regions should be considered to possibly have germ cell tumors. Serum (and tissue) markers should be obtained. Those chemotherapy regimens shown to be effective against testicular germ cell tumors may also be effective against these tumors.

THYROID CANCER

1. Thyroid cancer accounts for 0.2% of cancer deaths. However, occult carcinomas are found in 5–7% of autopsies and 10–15% of surgical thyroidectomy specimens. 30% occur in patients 30 years of age or younger.

2. The major types are:
   a. Follicular epithelium-papillary, papillary-follicular, follicular, Hürthle cell, anaplastic.
   b. Para-follicular cells-medullary carcinoma.
   c. Others (rare) lymphoma, sarcoma.

3. Some "pearls":
   a. Papillary carcinoma commonly invades lymphatics; follicular invades veins.
   b. Mixed papillary-follicular carcinomas are usually treated as papillary, but there is controversy about this.
   c. Medullary carcinomas (which account for 5–10%) may be sporadic or familial. When familial, they may be part of MEN-II syndrome (always check for pheo, too!).
   d. There is no agreed upon staging system.
   e. The presence of lymph node metastasis does not adversely affect prognosis.

4. Usually presents as neck mass felt by patient or palpated on routine exam. Local symptoms (e.g. pain, hoarseness) occur in 2.5% of cases.

5. Work up of a thyroid nodule:
   a. Thyroid scan—if "hot," not malignant; if "cold," may be (20% malignant); if "warm" nodule (i.e. overlying tissue gives some activity in nodule, treat as cold, i.e. R/O malignancy).

b. Ultrasound—cystic lesions rarely malignant.

c. Needle aspiration—very specific; false negative.

Evaluation of a Solitary Thyroid Nodule

d. If solid, can either aspirate, operate, or suppress and reevaluate in 6 months.

Strategies for following nodules with thyroid aspiration cytologies

1. Benign cytology
   Follow on or off L-T$_4$
   Growth on L-T$_4$—surgical biopsy
2. Malignant cytology—surgical biopsy

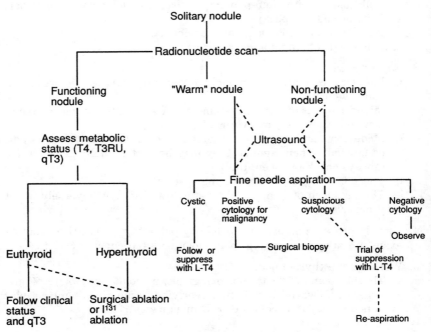

Figure 19.3

3. Inadequate cytology—repeat aspiration
4. Suspicious cytology
   Trial of L-T$_4$ for three months
   >50% regression—follow otherwise—surgical biopsy

6. Primary treatment
   a. For papillary or follicular cancers, total thyroidectomy is preferred (this is controversial, though). Prophylactic node dissection is not done.
   b. After thyroidectomy, follow with ^{131}I ablation.
   c. Then place on thyroid hormone replacement for life.
   d. For medullary carcinoma, total thyroidectomy is also treatment of choice, ^{131}I post operatively is not of benefit.
   e. Family members with MCT should be screened with baseline exams, calcitonin levels and some with provocative tests (e.g. pentagastrin stimulation). There is a premalignant lesion (C-cell hyperplasia) and removal of the thyroid when this is present is curative.
   f. For anaplastic cancer, surgery is the only effective therapy, but because of its rapid growth and tendency to invade, this is often impossible. Radiation may help.

7. For metastic disease
   a. ^{131}I may be useful, but the thyroid must be ablated, and the patient made avid for iodine (by becoming hypothyroid). ^{131}I can be used for scanning also. Uptake and effectiveness are correlated with the degree of differentiation of the cancer. Controlled trials of the effectiveness of the therapy are lacking.
   b. Consult the databases for the latest on chemotherapy.

UNKNOWN PRIMARY SITE CANCER

1. Between 1% and 9% of cancer patients present with metastatic cancer from an unknown primary site.
   It is uncertain why in some cases metastases may develop and become more prominent than the primary site.

2. Work-up includes a detailed history and complete physical examination (including pelvic and rectal exams). Epidemiologic risk factors, expo-

sures and family history are important. Be like Sherlock Holmes and don't dismiss any clue.

3. A key step is to discuss (beforehand if possible) with the pathologist what studies are most likely to be helpful (e.g. electron microscopy, markers, receptors, or special stains). Above the diaphragm, lung cancer is the most common obscure primary; below, pancreatic cancer is. In a woman, always consider breast cancer. Also, melanoma, kidney cancer and nasopharyngeal cancer are very "sneaky" in both sexes. Axillary carcinoma in a woman will usually be of breast origin. A squamous cell cancer arising in a neck node will usually be from head and neck area. A triple endoscopy should be done. Umbilical adenocarcinoma will most likely be a stomach primary. In a young man with a mediastinal mass, consider extragonadal germ cell tumors which are highly responsive to chemotherapy. (Measure serum and/or tissue levels of HCG and alphafetoprotein). Even at post-mortem examination the primary site is not identified in 15%.

4. Treatment:

If you can establish a diagnosis, do so and treat as you would that primary. Manage symptomatic local sites with radiation therapy or surgical excision. If squamous cell carcinoma in neck, treat as if head and neck metastasis with multidisciplinary approach. If male and <50, consider using a platinum based regimen in the event it may be of germ cell origin. If female, consider breast carcinoma as potential culprit, and using adoxorubicin based program for an empiric trial.

Chapter 20

Cancer Information Systems

More than perhaps any other medical subspecialty the field of medical oncology is involved with investigational forms of diagnosis and treatment. Cancer therapies move rapidly from bench to bedside and investigational therapies soon become state-of-the-art treatments. It is in this way that major strides in the conquest of cancer have occurred. Because these advances may be lifesaving if instituted in a timely fashion, it is important that the dissemination of oncologic information be as rapid as possible.

The widespread availability of the personal computer has made access to this expanding world of medical information easy, quick and inexpensive. Breakthroughs in technology, such as optical data storage, promise to make the process cheaper and even more simple in the future. Already, cancer information databases are being shared worldwide and, in the spirit of glasnost, the National Cancer Institute has made its databases PDQ and CANCERLIT available to Moscow, Warsaw, and Budapest. Unfortunately, many American house officers are still unfamiliar with the fascinating and helpful world of oncologic information available to them through the personal computer. The purpose of this chapter is to describe some of the tools and techniques available to students and housestaff for accessing the oncologic literature using the personal computer. Some of the basic hardware available to most housestaff and some of the more useful software and databases for oncology will be described.

A few basic computer terms should first be defined.

Modem: Short for modulator/demodulator. Device which couples two computers together over a normal voice telephone line allowing transmission of information.

Baud: The rate at which a modem can transmit or receive information. Equivalent to bits per second. A 2400 baud modem will transmit or receive roughly 240 characters per second.

Bit: Short for "binary digit." The most basic unit of information that a computer can store—either a 0 or a 1.

Byte: Eight bits of information which is enough to identify one character (a,b,c, etc.).

CD-ROM: Compact Disc-Read Only Memory. Optical storage medium able to store 550 megabytes.

Floppy: Short for floppy disk. A removable storage device holding magnetically coded information.

Hard Disk: A sealed device for storing large amounts of magnetically encoded information. Commonly contains between 20 and 200 megabytes of storage capacity.

Kilobyte: 1,024 bytes. Floppy disks often contain 400 to 800 K of storage capacity.

Megabyte: 1024 kilobytes or 1,048,576 bytes.

As technological advances, such as CD-ROM, become more prevalent, the method of accessing medical and oncologic literature is starting to change from one of remote computer access to direct searching of an optical compact disk.

The traditional and still widely used method of accessing a large reference database is to simply "call up" a central computer over an ordinary telephone line. This is done using a modem, which allows the personal computer to "talk" to the central "mainframe" computer. Information is then retrieved or "downloaded" to the personal computer and customarily printed out on paper as "hardcopy."

Any discussion of accessing medical literature is incomplete, however, without mentioning the role of the trained medical librarian. Medical librarians possess the knowledge to structure searches in a way that ensures maximal yield. This is most important when a manuscript is being prepared for publication or when a thorough bibliographic search on a topic is required. The use of an information specialist in this way is called "mediated searching." It is contrasted with "end-user" searching whereby the user is able to access the database on his/her own.

Almost every hospital medical library will have a personal computer and modem with the capability of downloading information from mainframe computers located at remote sites. This generally will be operated by a medical librarian who is familiar with the major databases commonly used by physicians. The librarian will be able to access MEDLINE at the National Library of Medicine (Bethesda, Maryland) and retrieve lists of articles and abstracts from the Cumulated Index Medicus. A search can be completed with a list of articles printed out in a very short time. The house officer can then review the printout and scan the appropriate articles in the hospital library. Alternatively, specific cancer information can be obtained through on-line access to the National Cancer Institute oncology database PDQ (Physician Data Query). This database is specifically designed for easy use by students, housestaff, and practitioners. It is menu-driven, making searches for information quite simple. Recently, NCI has made PDQ available to private vendors who are now marketing it as part of commercial on-line information services and on CD-ROM (see explanation below).

CD-ROM:Compact Disk-Read Only Memory
Essentially identical in concept to music CD. Cannot store new information.
Capable of also storing digitized graphics.
Can be read or "played" by IBM PC or Macintosh personal computers.
CD-ROM software is presently machine specific.

Requirements for On-Line System
Personal computer
Modem
Printer

Requirements for CD-ROM Based System
Personal computer
CD-ROM player
CD-ROM disk
Printer

Brief Description of the Most Frequently Used Oncology Databases

On-Line Searching
1) MEDLINE

Produced by National Library of Medicine.

Comprehensive database with seven million references—not oncology specific.

Equivalent to Index Medicus.

Articles from 1966 to present.

Updated monthly with 300,000 new articles added per year.

Provides list of references, most with abstracts.

May be searched on-line; special software known as GRATEFUL MED greatly facilitates access without the need for librarian assistance.

2) PHYSICIAN DATA QUERY (PDQ)

Produced by National Cancer Institute.

Oncology specific.

Menu driven for easy and intuitive searching by clinicians.

Requires no special training or computer experience.

Updated monthly by editorial board of experts.

Contains virtually all active clinical trials in USA and Canada.

Contains roster of cancer specialists by name and geographic area.

Contains staging, natural history, and treatment strategies for most adult and childhood malignancies.

Does give pertinent references to support treatment recommendations.

Contains a section written in simple language for distribution to patients and families.

Does not access MEDLINE to generate lists of articles or abstracts.

Is available on CD-ROM disk sold by private vendors and issued every 3 months.

Available on-line through NLM or through private vendors such as Compuserve.

Available on-line at Veterans Administration Hospitals.

3) KNOWLEDGE FINDER

CD-ROM system produced by Aries Systems Corporation for the Apple Macintosh.

Contains complete MEDLINE coverage.

Updated quarterly.

Each disk contains 300,000 references.

Uses artificial intelligence to enable searching without any special training.

Both general MEDLINE and oncology specific CANCERLIT disks available. CANCERLIT is a comprehensive collection of citations and abstracts of cancer literature from 3000 journals, papers, presentations, texts, and doctoral theses.

4) ONCODISC

A CD-ROM system product for the IBM-PC and compatible computer. Fully integrated oncology database on CD-ROM.

Issued in updated form every 3 months.

Contains most recent 3 years of CANCERLIT and PDQ as updated at time of disk release.

Contains complete oncology texts.

Cancer: Principles and Practice of Oncology (DeVita, et al), Important Advances in Oncology (Devita, et al) and Manual for Staging of Cancer (Beahrs/American Joint Committee on Cancer)

Clinical Applications and Examples

The following clinical situations demonstrate the usefulness of computer access for the house officer.

House officers are frequently presented with the necessity of "looking up current information" on cancer treatment. If there is a personal computer available with on-line access to PDQ, the search might proceed as follows. The initial screen as generally displayed on the PDQ menu is shown in Figure 20.1.

For a given problem it is very simple to follow the menu and select the appropriate area of the PDQ database to search. The screen shown is typical of PDQ in that you are given a series of numbered choices to select in order to obtain the needed information. As an example, if the patient in question has an unknown primary cancer with suspected brain metastases, the first selection would be #11 for Unknown Primary. One would then be shown the cancer diagnosis information retrieval menu as displayed here and could select #2, Summary for Physicians. This topic is covered by many "screens" of information but a representative one is displayed in Figure 20.2.

This screen discusses the natural history and most appropriate workup for carcinoma of unknown primary.

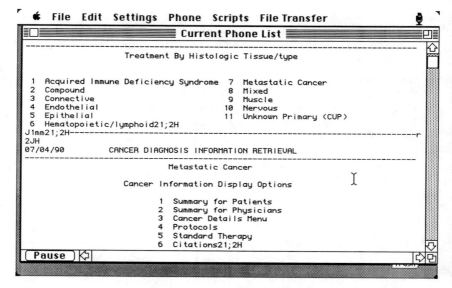

Figure 20.1.   Main PDQ menu screen.

If the patient is suffering from brain metastases and further information is sought, PDQ can provide information in the section of the database labeled #7 on the initial screen (Fig. 20.1). Shown in Figure 20.3 is the first screen from the section on state-of-the-art treatment of metastatic cancer.

The following screen displays more specific information about rain metastases, including signs, symptoms, and standard treatment approaches.

If information about experimental or research approaches to the treatment of a patient is sought, then PDQ can be utilized to display ongoing protocols that would seem to be appropriate for a given patient. This is reached through the PDQ protocol search menu. A representative screen is displayed in Figure 20.4 with the search having been "narrowed" to best fit the patient in question. A search for given protocols can be customized according to many different criteria, including type and stage of disease, type of therapy, and the patient's place of residence.

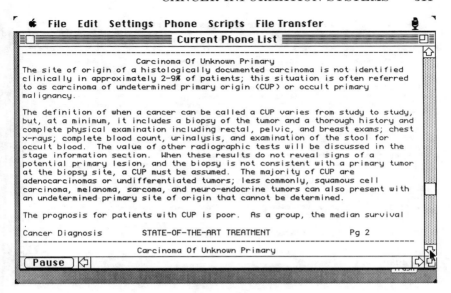

Figure 20.2.

If after studying a protocol the patient seemed appropriate for enrollment, PDQ would be able to display names, addresses and phone numbers of investigators participating in the study. This example points out the power of PDQ to provide state-of-the-art cancer information for house officers and to help with all phases of cancer diagnosis and treatment. Furthermore, it enables cancer specialists to make and receive appropriate patient referrals. Since cancer eligibility criteria are clearly outlined in the summary displayed by PDQ, it is relatively easy to refer patients to the most appropriate protocol for a specific situation. An additional and highly useful feature of PDQ is the Summary for Patients, which describes, in simple language, some of the more common malignancies and standard treatment options available. This can be printed out and given to the patient or family for reference. At present, this information is available only in English.

PDQ is not the only useful computerized oncology reference available to the house officer. Online access is becoming increasingly common in

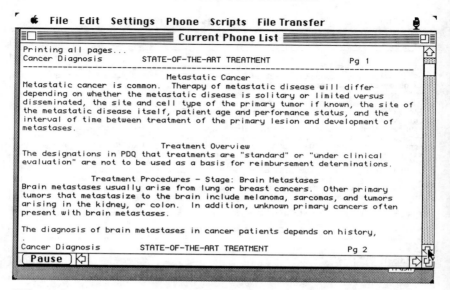

Figure 20.3. PDQ screen on state-of-the-art treatment of metastatic cancer.

hospitals and medical schools around the country. Summarized below are the names and phone numbers of major sources of computerized cancer information.

INFORMATION ABOUT COMPUTER DATABASES
National Library of Medicine
MEDLINE via GRATEFUL MED
SUBSCRIPTION INFORMATION 1-800-638-8480

BRS INFORMATION TECHNOLOGIES
Colleague MEDLINE via BRS/COLLEAGUE 1-800-289-4277
PAPERCHASE (617)-735-2253
Another user-friendly method of searching MEDLINE
ARIES SYSTEMS KNOWLEDGE FINDER (508)-475-7200

For those seeking further information on the dynamic field of medical computing contact:

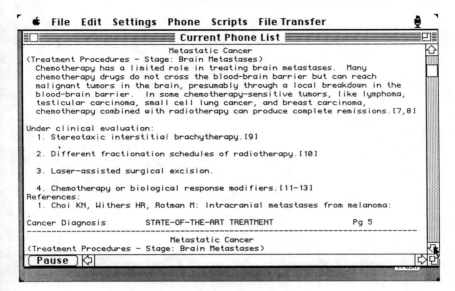

Figure 20.4.   PDQ protocol search menu.

American Medical Informatics Association
Suite 700
1101 Connecticut Avenue N.W.
Washington, D.C. 20036
Attn: Kitty Wyatt, Member Services
(202) 857-1189

Index

Page numbers followed by t or f indicate tables or figures, respectively. Page numbers in **boldface** indicate major discussions.